HEALTHFUL AGING

This new series is designed to meet the growing demand for current, accessible information about the increasingly popular wellness approach to personal health. The result of a collaborative effort by a highly professional writing, editorial, and publishing team, the *Wellness* series consists of 16 volumes, each on a single topic. Each volume in this attractively produced series combines original material with carefully selected readings, relevant statistical data, and illustrations. The series objectives are to increase awareness of the value of a wellness approach to personal health and to help the reader become a more informed consumer of health-related information. Employing a critical thinking approach, each volume includes a variety of assessment tools, discusses basic concepts, suggests key questions, and provides the reader with a list of resources for further exploration.

James K. Jackson	Wellness: AIDS, STD, & Other Communicable Diseases
Richard G. Schlaadt	Wellness: Alcohol Use & Abuse
Richard G. Schlaadt	Wellness: Drugs, Society, & Behavior
Robert E. Kime	Wellness: Environment & Health
Gary Klug & Janice Lettunich	Wellness: Exercise & Physical Fitness
James D. Porterfield & Richard St. Pierre	Wellness: Healthful Aging
Robert E. Kime	Wellness: The Informed Health Consumer
Paula F. Ciesielski	Wellness: Major Chronic Diseases
Robert E. Kime	Wellness: Mental Health
Judith S. Hurley	Wellness: Nutrition & Health
Robert E. Kime	Wellness: Pregnancy, Childbirth, & Parenting
David C. Lawson	Wellness: Safety & Accident Prevention
Randall R. Cottrell	Wellness: Stress Management
Richard G. Schlaadt	Wellness: Tobacco & Health
Randall R. Cottrell	Wellness: Weight Control
Judith S. Hurley & Richard G. Schlaadt	Wellness: The Wellness Life-Style

HEALTHFUL AGING

James D. Porterfield
Richard St. Pierre

WELLNESS

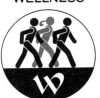

A MODERN
LIFE-STYLE
LIBRARY

The Dushkin Publishing Group, Inc./Sluice Dock, Guilford, CT 06437

Library of Congress Catalog Card Number: 91–057937
Manufactured in the United States of America
First Edition, First Printing
ISBN: 0–87967–866–6

Library of Congress Cataloging-in-Publication Data

Porterfield, James D., Healthful Aging (Wellness)
    1. Aging. 2. Health. I. St. Pierre, Richard. II. Title. III. Series.
RA773   612.67   91–057937   ISBN 0–87967–866–6

Please see page 146 for credits.

The procedures and explanations given in this publication are based on
research and consultation with medical and nursing authorities. To the best
of our knowledge, these procedures and explanations reflect currently
accepted medical practice; nevertheless, they cannot be considered absolute
and universal recommendations. For individual application, treatment
suggestions must be considered in light of the individual's health, subject to
a doctor's specific recommendations. The authors and the publisher disclaim
responsibility for any adverse effects resulting directly or indirectly from the
suggested procedures, from any undetected errors, or from the reader's
misunderstanding of the text.

JAMES D. PORTERFIELD

James D. Porterfield brings to his work a useful combination of experience and talents. Currently an instructor in the Division of Continuing Education at the Pennsylvania State University, he is also a freelance writer specializing in high-school and college-level educational materials. In addition to *Healthful Aging,* he has published 2 previous books and is at work on another.

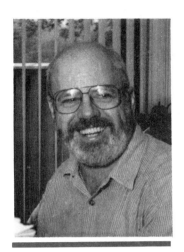

RICHARD ST. PIERRE

Richard St. Pierre is a professor in the Department of Health Education at the Pennsylvania State University, where he has served as department head since 1978. He received his master's degree in public health from UCLA and his doctorate from the University of North Carolina, where he served as an assistant professor prior to his appointment at Penn State. His major research interests are changes in health behavior across the lifespan and the factors that influence those changes. In addition to *Healthful Aging,* he is the author of over 50 articles and co-author of a human sexuality textbook and an elementary health education series for grades 3–8.

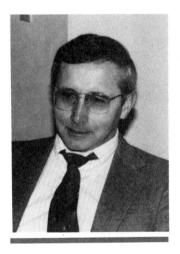

WELLNESS:
A Modern Life-Style Library

General Editors
Robert E. Kime, Ph.D.
Richard G. Schlaadt, Ed.D.

Authors
Paula F. Ciesielski, M.D.
Randall R. Cottrell, Ed.D.
Judith S. Hurley, M.S., R.D.
James K. Jackson, M.D.
Robert E. Kime, Ph.D.
Gary A. Klug, Ph.D.
David C. Lawson, Ph.D.
Janice Lettunich, M.S.
James D. Porterfield
Richard St. Pierre, Ph.D.
Richard G. Schlaadt, Ed.D.

Developmental Staff
Irving Rockwood, Program Manager
Paula Edelson, Series Editor
Wendy Connal, Administrative Assistant
Jason J. Marchi, Editorial Assistant

Editing Staff
John S. L. Holland, Managing Editor
Janet M. Jamilkowski, Copy Editor
Diane Barker, Editorial Assistant
Mary L. Strieff, Art Editor
Robert Reynolds, Illustrator

Production and Design Staff
Brenda S. Filley, Production Manager
Whit Vye, Cover Design and Logo
Jeremiah B. Lighter, Text Design
Libra Ann Cusack, Typesetting Supervisor
Charles Vitelli, Designer
Meredith Scheld, Graphics Assistant
Steve Shumaker, Graphics Assistant
Lara M. Johnson, Graphics Assistant
Juliana Arbo, Typesetter
Richard Tietjen, Editorial Systems Analyst

AGING IS A UNIVERSAL process. It happens to each of us from the moment of birth. And yet aging as an experience is unique to each individual. It is not an illness. It is not something to be cured.

Although aging and death may be inevitable, physical disability and a declining health status during our later years are not. Nor are mental confusion or senility, inactivity, and a dependency on others. These debilitating conditions are brought on by our heredity, environment, and life-style. Our health and vigor is something we can influence, even in old age. Increasingly, research is showing that many conditions once thought to be the consequence of aging are in fact the result of disease. We are learning that a healthy life-style and a wellness approach to aging can forestall such diseases and allow us to arrive at death's doorstep having led a vigorous, joyful, and productive life through all our years.

Throughout, mention is made of both those aspects of aging over which you exercise some control and those over which you exercise little control. In the former instance you can take steps to forestall the aging process. This book is predicated on the belief that, by increasing your understanding of the aging process, and by exploring the ways in which you can manage it, you can overcome any fears you may have about aging. Better yet, you can increase the length and quality of the life you have. Special attention is paid to key concepts such as physical fitness, sound nutrition, and stress management. You are urged to commit to a plan of action tailored to your own situation and goals, and tips are provided to help you stick to your plan.

This is not a definitive work, but rather a place to begin. The central objective of this book is not to make you into an instant expert on aging but to help you learn to *think critically* about this universal process. Only then will you be able to distinguish aging fact from aging myth, and only then will you be an informed health consumer.

James D. Porterfield
Richard St. Pierre
State College, PA

Contents

1

Growing Older: The Aging Process

Page 1

2

Aging and Its Physical Consequences

Page 21

6

Influencing the Aging Process

Page 110

FIGURES

TABLES

Growing Older: The Aging Process

"Your body is, in a sense, a business of which you are the sole proprietor."

—Isadore Rossman

DOES THIS SOUND familiar? The day begins early with a brief warm-up, then out the door for a half-hour of brisk exercise. Back home, breakfast is followed with a shower, dressing for work, and getting on the road before traffic gets heavy. At the Chamber of Commerce, the day is spent on the telephone, in meetings, and conducting visits to customers, either to sell advertising space in the Chamber's monthly magazine or to arrange exhibitors at the annual convention. Every day seems to present new and interesting challenges and responsibilities. Work is interrupted by lunch with old friends in town for the week. The day ends with classes at a local university, completing courses needed for a degree. Course work has to be completed by spring because marriage lies just ahead: the wedding is set for May. At day's end, a sense of exhaustion sets in, as does a feeling of satisfaction at what has been accomplished.

This may be you. At age 75!

A number of significant developments have increased the likelihood that you will live into your 90s, perhaps beyond. New medical successes have brought childhood diseases under effective control or eliminated them altogether, resulting in a marked decline in deaths during childhood. The chances of surviving the life-threatening hazards of youth, too, are greater now than ever

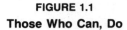

FIGURE 1.1
Those Who Can, Do

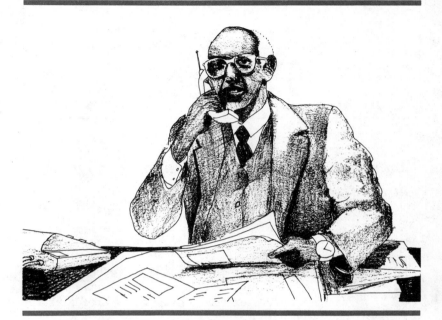

Old age does not mean being "put out to pasture." As of 1989, approximately 3.4 million older Americans were in the labor force—2 million men and 1.4 million women.

before. In 1900, for example, one person in 4 died before the age of 20. Today only one out of 50 newborns dies before its 20th birthday. [1]

As you approach adulthood, other factors work to further increase the number of years you can expect to live. These include a more informed approach to diet and nutrition; improvements in the environment and in public sanitation; advances in surgical techniques and drugs, as well as in the ability to identify and provide early treatment of chronic illnesses and infectious diseases; and the slow but steady decline in cigarette smoking. As a result of all these developments, you can expect to live substantially longer than your grandparents.

This increase in life expectancy makes it appropriate and necessary for you to consider and prepare now for your later

FIGURE 1.2
Average Life Expectancy, 1900–1990

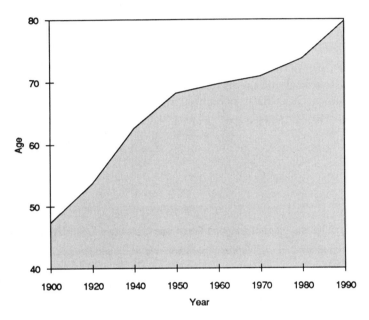

Source: Department of Health and Human Services.

Average life expectancy at birth in the United States reached a record high in 1990. This continues the upward trend in life expectancy since the beginning of the century. The greatest gains occurred between 1900 and 1950 and were largely due to dramatic reductions in deaths from infectious diseases.

years. Most of us, however, are uncomfortable thinking about aging, for a number of reasons. First, we think of aging as a process of decline, not of growth. Second, the unavoidable outcome of aging is death, which is unpleasant for us to contemplate at any time. Finally, there are many myths that surround aging and cloud our ability to think of it positively.

These attitudes and falsehoods should not deter you from thinking seriously about how you want to live as you grow older. If you want to enjoy the freedom, experiences, and rewards that your old age will hold for you, and to meet the challenges as well, it is wise to begin today to prepare yourself both physically and mentally for that time. You should begin this preparation by first setting aside some of the myths about aging that are prevalent in our culture today.

MYTHS AND FACTS ABOUT AGING AND ELDERS

Many think of old age as a time of sickness and disability; loneliness and depression; frailty and dependence; forgetfulness, confusion, and senility; poor health; physical inactivity and sexual inadequacy. If you hold these views, *you are mistaken.*

Where do such myths originate? In part, they are a carryover from earlier times. Until recently, the human life span was a

Table 1.1 Life Expectancy at Birth for Selected Countries, 1987

	Male	Female
Japan	75.9	82.1
Sweden	74.2	80.4
Switzerland	74.0	81.0
Canada	73.3	80.2
Cuba	73.0	76.5
France	72.6	81.1
England and Wales	72.6	78.3
Kuwait	72.5	75.8
United States	71.5	78.4
Singapore	71.3	76.5
Chile	70.0	75.7
Czechoslovakia	67.7	75.3
Poland	66.8	75.2
U.S.S.R.	65.1	73.9

Source: Adapted from Department of Health and Human Services, *Health United States*, 1990, pp. 74–75.

While average life expectancy in the United States has increased dramatically since 1900, some other nations have done even better. In virtually all nations for which reliable data is available, however, women outlive men. The reported differences range from as little as 3 years (Kuwait) to almost 9 years (U.S.S.R.).

relatively short one; a person born in 1890 could expect to live to be 42. [2] Today, however, 1 in 3 men and one half of all women born in 1988 can expect to live nearly twice as long, to 80. [3] By the time today's newborn babies in the United States reach the age of 20, their life expectancy may approach 85 years. Nonetheless, we still retain images of what life will be like as an elder from the days when old age set in at around the 40th year. And before today's emphasis on health and fitness made possible a vigorous later life, that earlier "old age" was more likely to have consisted of early and longer-lasting signs of physical or mental decline.

Another strong influence on our thinking is the media, which so often celebrates youth and portrays older people as unhealthy, unstylish, and uninteresting. [4] That these impressions are based on untrue assumptions or upon conditions that can be easily corrected seems not to prevent the creators of such messages from perpetuating myths about aging.

The fact is, older adults today are healthier, more active, and more involved than they have ever been before. They also have a wider range of life-style options than at any previous time. Furthermore, we can expect these trends to continue.

It's time then to reconsider many of the myths we harbor about old age. Among these are the following:

1. Myth: *Old age is a time of sickness and disability.*
Fact: Among the 95 percent of older Americans not living in a health-care institution, only 2 percent are confined to bed most of the day by some form of chronic condition. Another 7 percent need help getting around in and outside their neighborhoods. The remaining 86 percent are not seriously impaired by health problems.

2. Myth: *Old age is marked by loneliness and depression.*
Fact: While certain life-style changes—such as retirement, the death of a spouse, a child, or a friend—may lead to loneliness or depression, very few elders are truly alone. Over 80 percent of older Americans have children or other relatives living nearby with whom they have daily contact. In all, approximately 9.5 million—or 82 percent—of older men, and 9.3 million—or 57 percent—of older women live in families. [5] Almost two thirds of all Americans aged 65 and older vote in each election. Almost one fourth report that they devote time and energy to volunteer work in their communities.

(continued on p. 11)

A Fact Quiz on Aging

T F   1. Everyone becomes "senile" sooner or later if he or she lives long enough.

T F   2. All five of your senses tend to decline in old age.

T F   3. Most people over the age of 60 have no interest in or capacity for sexual activity.

T F   4. At least one half of all old people live in long-term care institutions, such as nursing homes, mental hospitals, homes for the aged, and the like.

T F   5. Most old people are set in their ways and unable to change.

T F   6. Personality changes with age, just like hair gets grey and skin wrinkles.

T F   7. More women than men survive to old age.

T F   8. Once you reach old age, you no longer have to be concerned about calcium for strong bones and teeth.

T F   9. As you grow older, you need more vitamins and minerals to stay healthy.

T F   10. Mental confusion is an inevitable, incurable consequence of old age.

T F   11. If you have been smoking for 30 or 40 years, it does you no good to quit.

T F   12. Most older women are widows, while most older men are married.

T F   13. Your intelligence declines as you grow old.

T F   14. Old people usually take longer to learn something new.

T F   15. Physical strength tends to decline in old age.

T F   16. Most older workers are not as effective at their work as younger workers.

T F   17. The reaction time of most older people tends to be slower than the reaction time of younger people.

T F   18. The majority of older people have incomes below the poverty level as defined by the federal government.

Answer Key: 1. False; 2. True; 3. False; 4. False; 5. False; 6. False; 7. True; 8. False; 9. False; 10. False; 11. False; 12. True; 13. False; 14. False; 15. True; 16. False; 17. True; 18. False.

Source: "What Is Your Aging IQ?" *National Institute on Aging* (Washington, 1986), p. 1.

Old Age Is Not What It Used to Be

Age only matters when one is aging. Now that I have arrived at a great age, I might as well be 20.

—*Pablo Picasso (at 80)*

Adult life used to be fairly predictable, and so were theories of aging. It was simple: the older you got, the more you lost—sex drive, memory, brain cells, energy, intelligence. When psychologists first studied adult development, they would come around every few years and draw conclusions about the inevitable losses associated with age. Now they come around every few years and find that Grandma refuses to mind the grandchildren; she and Harry have bought a Winnebago and are camping in Yosemite. Aunt Sarah took up marathon running and local politics at the age of 73. And Uncle Fred retired at 58 from Amalgamated Teabiscuit & Muffins to become a jazz musician. Growing old is not what it used to be.

No one even agrees anymore on what "old" is. Not long ago, 30 was middle-aged and 60 was old. Now, more and more people are living into their 70's, 80's and beyond—and many of them are living well, without any incapacitating mental or physical decline. Today, old age is defined not simply by chronological years, but by degree of health and well-being.

I realized how my ideas of "old" had changed when I began looking for people to interview for this story. My friends who are in their 70's—such as Anne Louis, a 75-year-old realtor who worked night and day for months to find a house for my husband and me—were too young. Those in their 80's, like my mother, were busy working, exercising, traveling and fund raising; they didn't seem properly old either. And when I asked around for names of vigorous, interesting people in their 90's, I had more than I could manage within a day.

Until recently, people believed that all mental and physical functions declined with age. "Old" meant forgetful, senile and feeble. But many researchers are now finding that some of the conditions thought characteristic of old age are a result of poor nutrition, lack of exercise or disease, such as Alzheimer's and other neurologically based dementias. According to Dr. T. Franklin Williams, director of the National Institute on Aging, even the heart and kidneys of a person over 65, if free of disease, can function as well as those of a young person.

In separating the biology of aging from its psychology, researchers have begun to realize that many of the presumed psychological deficits of old age would occur to people of any age who were deprived of loved ones, close friends, meaningful activity and intellectual stimulation.

When people don't lose these necessities, they often end up like Luba Kahan, who just turned 90 and has every marble she was born with. She did quit smoking last year because her children were pestering her about it, and she once took a "poison" prescribed by her doctor for a backache, but she continues to horrify her 73-year-old son by eating what she likes rather than what she should. "My philosophy," she explains, "is that as long as you don't see a doctor, you'll stay healthy. When my son is as old as I am, he can tell me what to eat." Mrs. Kahan lives alone, walks to the local supermarket, reads all night when it suits her and continues to be busy and independent. "The only thing I need from my children," she says, "is love."

Many of the assumptions about mental and physical decline in old age were based on studies that compared several age groups and that did not distinguish between aging itself and the effects of illness, poverty, poor education or lack of intellectual stimulation. Although these studies found that some aspects of intelligence, such as reasoning ability, spatial ability and verbal comprehension, declined with age, more recent work, which followed the same people from middle age into old age, showed far less decline. This has led researchers to re-evaluate the earlier findings and question whether a decrease in mental abilities is natural to old age or whether it is specific to generational cohorts, people who have shared certain experiences and problems.

"Each aging group is different because of its particular history," says Dr. Jacqueline Good-childs, associate professor of psychology at the University of California at Los Angeles and a researcher at the RAND Corporation. "Gerontology is a fascinating field because you know the findings will change every five years. For example, the average retirement age is now under 60. A whole generation is starting over at 59, finding new careers and interests." Dr. Goodchilds and her research associate, Leonie Huddy, even suspect that osteoporosis is a generational artifact—characteristic of a cohort of older women who, as young girls, rarely exercised and did not develop full bone strength.

According to Dr. Goodchilds, the generation now in their 40's and 50's "will be yet a different breed of old people—they are better educated, they have more skills."

"Many more of them are single and childless, and they worry about growing old on their own," she adds. "But we've found that in old age, never-married people report much higher life satisfaction than widowed people do, perhaps because they are used to doing things on their own. They do not experience the discontinuity that married people do when the spouse dies or the children move away."

"Old people in general feel psychologically better than young people," says Dr. Carin Rubenstein, a social psychologist and co-author, with Dr. Phillip Shaver, of "In Search of Intimacy," a study of loneliness in America. "They have fewer worries about themselves and how they look to other people; they have higher self-esteem; they aren't as lonely as people think they are." The loneliest people, Dr. Rubenstein says, are not the elderly, but teen-agers and young adults.

Young people just starting out in new careers and relationships are also under far more stress than older people, and have less experience in coping with it. This is one reason that many experts are now celebrating some of the benefits of aging: wisdom, a sense of humor, old-fashioned maturity.

The effort to distinguish biological changes from psychological consequences has begun to erode many of the stereotypes of age. For instance, until recently it was assumed that the menopausal woman suffered from a syndrome that made her deeply depressed about losing her reproductive capacity, her sexuality, her femininity. This stereotype evolved chiefly from studies of women whose early menopause was brought on by surgery and from the assumption that women *naturally* become depressed when their reproductive capacity ends. Actually, most women go through normal menopause with no major psychological difficulties and very few physical ones.

Drs. Sonja McKinlay and John McKinlay, at the Cambridge Research Center in Cambridge, Mass., surveyed more than 8,000 menopausal women. Only 3 percent said they felt regret; the majority viewed menopause with relief, or had no particular feelings about it at all, apart from annoyance at such "temporarily bothersome symptoms" as hot flashes and menstrual irregularity. "If the truth were known," says Dr. Goodchilds, "we'd have to diagnose them as having P.M.F.—Post-Menstrual Freedom."

Certainly, aging produces physical limitations, as any 32-year-old "aging" athlete knows. The body generally reaches its peak condition at about age 30 and then slowly declines. Eyesight gets worse; it becomes more difficult, particularly for men, to hear tones in the higher registers; the sense of smell weakens after age 65 and drops sharply after age 80; the central nervous system processes information more slowly than it once did, and metabolism and reflexes slow down.

Yet aging does not inevitably mean the loss of intelligence or memory. Folklore has it that the brain loses brain cells the way the scalp sheds dandruff, but according to Dr. Marian Diamond, professor of anatomy at the University of California at Berkeley, normal human aging does not produce extensive brain cell deterioration until, perhaps, extreme old age. From her research with aged rats, and with vigorous, healthy people over the age of 88, Dr. Diamond is optimistic about the brain's "plasticity"—the ability of nerve cells to respond to stimuli—at any age. When people live in challenging environments, she argues, brain function does not naturally decay.

A case in point is Scott O'Dell, 89, who has written at least one book every year since 1966. His research has taken him to Bermuda, the Yucatan, Guatemala, Peru and the Pacific Northwest. He was 62 when his first children's book, "Island of the Blue Dolphins," was published.

Mr. O'Dell holds no truck with live-right-to-live-long theories. "There's no secret to being 89," he says. "No regimen, no trick, such as eating Wheaties, jogging 10 miles a day, drinking alcohol, not drinking alcohol. There is only the great, overriding secret: it all amounts to genes. My Irish great-great-grandfather died at 105. He was perfectly healthy at the time, but he fell off the porch. Drunk, I'm sure. He had 11 sons, and even counting the one who died at 36, their average age when they died was 96. Maybe I have a few of those genes."

Genes are helpful, Dr. Diamond agrees, but they are not sufficient. "A nerve cell is designed to receive stimuli," she explains. "Without stimuli, it shrivels and decays. This is true of the rat brain and the human brain, the young brain and the old brain. I've known many people with long-lived parents who died young, unhappy and unfulfilled. And I've known people whose genes were against them who have lived long, healthy lives."

It's not a matter of diet versus genes, or heredity versus environment, Dr. Diamond says; it's how they interact. "My father lived to be 93," she says. "He ate an egg every day, but he had low cholesterol. People scream about cholesterol without knowing their own levels. The important thing is to know yourself."

A healthy old age, everyone agrees, depends on activity. Not only are older adults just as good as young ones at long-practiced abilities, they can also acquire new ones. In a study published in 1986, Dr. K. Warner Schaie, director of the gerontology center at Pennsylvania State University, and Dr. Sherry Willis of the department of human development at Penn State, were able to reverse the supposedly normal intellectual decline in a group of 60- to 80-year-olds by giving each of them five one-hour tutoring sessions in inductive reasoning and problem solving.

As for the universal fear of memory loss, it appears that memory plays tricks on everyone. I don't know one person over the age of 25 who hasn't complained about his or her lousy memory, or made nervous jokes about having Alzheimer's. The short-term memory of most older people—the ability to remember the name of a person they just met or a phone number they just looked up—is not much different from that of most younger people. It is long-term memory that tends to cause problems. But according to one recent study, years of schooling and current enrollment in school are better predictors of differences in memory ability than age is.

"Old people get bored taking boring tests," says Dr. Goodchilds. "A young person who is used to frequent school exams will sit still for four hours, counting numbers backward, if you ask him to. An older person will say, 'What the hell am I doing here?' "

As Dr. Robin West, a psychologist at the University of Florida at Gainesville, observes, most memory studies do not take place in the real world. It is important to remember to call your doctor or pay your bills, but it isn't important to remember nonsense syllables. When the material is relevant to them, older people can retrieve information as rapidly as younger people can. If they do have trouble remembering something, the reason seems to be slower reaction time, not impaired recall. In other words, we all eventually come up with the name of the actor who starred with Dustin Hoffman in "Midnight Cowboy"; it just takes some of us a little longer.

Perhaps the biggest difference between an old person and a young person who can't remember something is that the former can blame forgetfulness on old age. When my mother, who remembers more about my life than I do, can't think of a name immediately, she says, "Damn, I'm getting old." When my 19-year-old students can't remember the answer to a test question, they just say "Damn."

As with intelligence and memory, a decline in the frequency of sexual activity among older people is, researchers suspect, due less to biology than to social and psychological factors, including the *expectation* of such a decline.

Aging does cause some physiological changes in sexual response—women produce less vaginal lubrication, men take longer to reach full erection, and both sexes have fewer contractions at orgasm—but these changes do not necessarily affect frequency of sexual activity or pleasure. The main problem for most old people is lack of a partner, not lack of desire.

The frequency of a person's sexual experiences in early adulthood is the best predictor of his or her sexual activity in later life. According to Dr. Carole Wade, a psychologist and author of "Human Sexuality," "The greatest difference in sexual activity—or any other aspect of aging—is not between the old and the young, but between individuals."

This emphasis on individual development, and the corresponding move away from "stage-oriented" approaches, is perhaps the most dramatic change in theories of aging. "Unlike child development, which is powerfully governed by maturational and biological changes, adult development is more affected by psychology and experience," observes Dr. Orville Brim, a social psychologist and member of the MacArthur Foundation's Program of Successful Aging, a national committee of 15 experts from different fields. "This means that so-called adult stages cannot be as universal or as inevitable as childhood stages. Children go through a stage of babbling before they talk, they crawl before they walk. But as children mature, environmental factors take on greater impact. That's why you find far more variation among 80-year-olds than among 8-year-olds."

Many researchers are now turning their attention to the transitions that mark adulthood. What matters, they say, is not how old you are, but what you are doing.

"Having a child affects new parents regardless of *when* they have a child," says Dr. Nancy Schlossberg, a developmental psychologist at the University of Maryland. "People facing retirement confront similar issues whether they are retiring at 40, 50 or 70. Adolescents may have identity problems, but so do adult auto workers who are laid off and divorced homemakers who must find new careers."

Unlike stage theories, which assume that life consists of a series of psychological crises that must be resolved before an individual can move on, transition theories assume that all human beings have certain psychological needs that can never be satisfied once and for all, but must be constantly renegotiated. To Dr. Schlossberg, these needs include a reasonable degree of control over one's life, enthusiasm for one's activities and commitments to people and values. Most of all, she says, people need to feel that they *matter* to others.

To see Dr. Schlossberg's theory in the flesh, you should meet Benjamin Rosen, a 92-year-old musician who single-handedly runs a sheet music shop in Hollywood. Mr. Rosen turns every visiting questioner into a straight man. (*Do you still play?* No, I actively play. *What do you play?* Violin, viola, pinochle. . . .) When I ask him how long he has had the store and whether he ever plans to retire, he says, "I don't have the store; the store has me. People rely on me. As a musician, I know what they need. Look at this picture of my kid brother. He's 65 and retired. I'm 92 and working. Who's better off?"

To Marian Diamond, there's no contest. "Having taught anatomy all these years," she says, "I always go back to the heart. It is designed by evolution to look after itself first, and then the rest of the body. This is not selfishness, but wisdom; when people feel good about themselves, they are able to give to others."

"I firmly believe that love is essential to a healthy old age—love of oneself and the ability to love someone besides oneself."

"Can a person change late in life?" I ask.

"You can change nerve cells at any age," says Dr. Diamond. "You just need the right environment."

Source: Carol Tavris, *New York Times Magazine,* 27 September 1987, pp. 24–25, 91–92.

FIGURE 1.3
And They Haven't Given Up on Politics Either

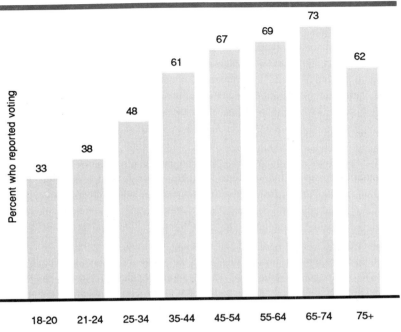

Source: Bureau of the Census, Current Population Reports, 1989.

In 1988 almost 20 million (19 percent) of the 102 million Americans who reported voting in that year's election were 65 years old or older. Although voting tends to decline over the age of 75, it increases steadily up to that point with those in the 55–64 and 65–74 age groups being the most likely to vote.

3. Myth: *Old people are frail and dependent.*
Fact: Only 5 percent of older Americans live in nursing homes or other closely supervised health-care facilities. The other 95 percent live basically healthy and independent lives. Nearly 80 percent have and live in their own homes. In fact, the percentage of people aged 18 to 34 living at home with their parents is greater than the percentage of people over 60 who live with a younger relative.
4. Myth: *Old people are forgetful, confused, and senile.*
Fact: Only 20 to 25 percent of those who live to be 80 or older

develop Alzheimer's disease or some other form of degenerative brain disease. While we often assume that these are the only possible sources of forgetfulness and confusion, such symptoms can result from more than 100 causes, such as a minor head injury, a high fever, poor nutrition, or an adverse reaction to a medicine. Such things can happen to anyone—no matter at what **chronological age**—and are not unique to older adults. In addi-

What do you mean when you describe someone as "old"? Truth is, there is no precise age at which a person becomes "old." Some people are "old" at 25; others are still young at 75.

There were times, even in the United States, when old age began in one's thirties; around 1900, for instance, when life expectancy was about 47. Today most younger people define old age as "somewhere

Coming to Terms: Defining "Old"

in the sixties." When they get to their sixties, however, people tend to define "old" as "ten years older than I." In the not too distant future, people won't be described as "old" until they are in their 80s or 90s.

In fact, as Simone de Beauvoir notes in *The Coming of Age*, there is no initiation ceremony into old age; it can be anywhere from 50 to 90. "Old" is not automatically a matter of birthdays, for there are health and psychological factors. "You're as old as you feel" is a familiar axiom. By such criteria, a rule-of-thumb definition of old age might be: when a person is no longer capable of carrying on or living independently. That is not, of course, an exact or totally accurate measure; but it has the virtue of suggesting an *individual* assessment.

The alternative, based on society's attitudes, is general and automatic, making people old by the numbers, whether 60 years, 65, or even 70. It is what Maggie Kuhn of the Gray Panthers, among others, refers to as "sociogenic aging": the role society imposes on people at a certain chronological age. More saddening is the extent to which older people themselves are sometimes brainwashed into accepting such a role. They learn that they are supposed to "act their age," and they act that way. They may accept the myth that aging leads to incompetence and forget that people like Michelangelo and Goethe, Einstein and Edison, and many others, achieved great work in their sixties, seventies, and eighties.

Each of us will have to learn to judge productivity, not chronological age. Old age is just another phase in the life cycle to once again "repot" the plant that has outgrown its container.

Source: Irving R. Dickman, *Ageism: Discrimination Against Older People* (New York: Public Affairs Committee, Inc., 1979), 6.

Chronological age: The actual length of time that a person has lived, usually measured in years.

tion, the root causes of such symptoms are often curable. [6] A person's **mental age** is to a significant degree based on his or her attitude.

5. Myth: *Old age is accompanied by poor health.*
Fact: Surveys find that fewer than one in 5 older Americans consider themselves to be in poor health.

6. Myth: *Old age is a time of physical inactivity.*
Fact: If this is true, it is by choice and not necessity. Many older people both enjoy and benefit from regular exercise. Especially popular forms of exercise include bicycling, swimming, and walking. So a person's **biological age** does *not* automatically imply an inability to be physically active.

7. Myth: *Old people are sexually inadequate.*
Fact: A person's level of sexual activity in old age tends to reflect his or her level of such activity in earlier years. Those most sexually active during youth and middle age will continue to be the most sexually active as senior citizens. Most older people can, and do, lead active and satisfying sex lives. [7]

These are but a sample of the many myths and stereotypes that many of us hold about old age. Small wonder that we often find it difficult even to contemplate, let alone plan for, our later years. The first step in remedying this situation is to recognize such beliefs for what they are, myths. The next is to take a new and more realistic look at old age, its realities, its hazards, and its rewards.

WHY BE CONCERNED WITH AGING?

There are several reasons why you should know about and understand the **aging process**. First, it is a process that all of us experience throughout our lives. As living organisms, all of us experience to varying degrees the effects of the aging process on a daily basis. Furthermore, as living organisms, we will, if our lives are full, experience 3 more or less distinct phases during our **life span**. The first phase, **maturation**, is characterized by growth and development. The second phase, **maturity**, is the interval during which our skills and abilities are at their peak. Finally, during the **aging** phase, we experience a gradual decline in many of our physical and some of our mental abilities.

Mental age: A person's level of intellectual functioning regardless of his or her chronological age; generally attributed to the French psychologist Alfred Binet (1857–1911).

Biological age: A person's age as determined by his or her overall physiological condition, expressed as the chronological age for which that condition is regarded as typical or average.

Aging process: The ongoing series of regular and generally predictable changes in physical and mental condition that accompany an increase in chronological age.

Life span: The interval between birth and death, which may be divided into 3 more or less distinct phases—maturation, maturity, and aging.

Maturation: The first stage of the life cycle, during which physical growth is completed, much learning takes place, and physical and mental abilities and skills reach their peak stage of development.

Maturity: The second stage of the life cycle, during which learning continues and physical and mental skills and abilities are maintained at a peak or near-peak stage of development.

Aging: The third and final stage of the life cycle, characterized by a continuation of learning, accompanied by a decline—at varying rates—in physical and mental skills and abilities.

FIGURE 1.4
The Aging of America

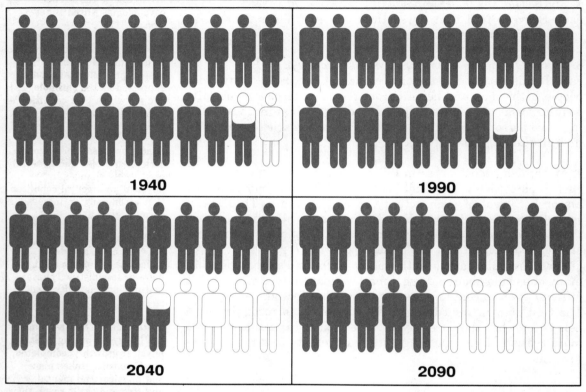

Source: *FDA Consumer,* October 1988.

In 1990 approximately 12.7 percent of the U.S. population was 65 or older, in comparison with only 6.8 percent in 1940. It is estimated that older Americans will account for over one-fifth (21.7 percent) of the total U.S. population by 2040, and one-fourth of the population by 2090.

This process, however, should not be thought of as a one-way street. Getting older does not inevitably mean decline. We are all in a state of continual development and change. As an infant, each of us possesses talents—the seemingly effortless ability to put our toes in our mouth, for example—that have long since disappeared even by the time we enter kindergarten. Similarly, our ability to learn reaches its maximum in at least some areas during our early childhood years, as any adult who has attempted

(continued on p. 17)

Calculating Your Life Expectancy

How many more years can you expect to live? For an estimate, consult the following table, which is based upon 1986 data from the National Center for Health Statistics.

Age	All races		Whites		Other Races		Age	All races		Whites		Other Races	
	M	F	M	F	M	F		M	F	M	F	M	F
At birth	71.3	78.3	72.0	78.8	67.2	75.1	38	36.4	42.1	36.8	42.4	33.5	39.7
1	71.1	78.0	71.7	78.4	67.4	75.1	39	35.5	41.1	35.9	41.5	32.5	38.7
2	70.2	77.0	70.8	77.5	66.4	74.2	40	34.5	40.2	34.9	40.5	31.8	37.8
3	69.2	76.1	69.8	76.5	65.5	73.2							
4	68.2	75.1	68.8	75.5	64.5	72.3	41	33.6	39.2	34.0	39.6	31.0	36.9
5	67.3	74.1	67.8	74.6	63.6	71.3	42	32.8	38.3	33.1	38.6	30.2	36.0
6	66.3	73.1	66.9	73.6	62.6	70.3	43	31.9	37.3	32.2	37.7	29.4	35.1
7	65.3	72.2	65.9	72.6	61.6	69.4	44	31.0	36.4	31.3	36.7	28.6	34.3
8	64.3	71.2	64.9	71.6	60.6	68.4	45	30.1	35.5	30.4	35.8	27.8	33.4
9	63.3	70.2	63.9	70.6	59.7	67.4	46	29.2	34.6	29.5	34.9	27.0	32.5
10	62.4	69.2	62.9	69.6	58.7	66.4	47	28.4	33.7	28.7	33.9	26.2	31.6
							48	27.5	32.8	27.8	33.0	25.4	30.8
11	61.4	68.2	61.9	68.6	57.7	65.4	49	26.6	31.8	26.9	32.1	24.6	29.9
12	60.4	67.2	61.0	67.7	56.7	64.4	50	25.8	31.0	26.1	31.2	23.9	29.1
13	59.4	66.2	60.0	66.7	55.7	63.4							
14	58.4	65.2	59.0	65.7	54.8	62.5	51	25.0	30.1	25.2	30.3	23.1	28.2
15	57.5	64.3	58.0	64.7	53.8	61.5	52	24.1	29.2	24.4	29.4	22.4	27.4
16	56.5	63.3	57.1	63.7	52.8	60.5	53	23.3	28.3	23.6	28.6	21.7	26.6
17	55.6	62.3	56.1	62.8	51.9	59.5	54	22.5	27.5	22.7	27.7	21.0	25.8
18	54.6	61.3	55.2	61.8	51.0	58.6	55	21.8	26.6	21.9	26.8	20.3	25.0
19	53.7	60.4	54.3	60.8	50.0	57.6	56	21.0	25.8	21.2	26.0	19.6	24.2
20	52.8	59.4	53.4	59.9	49.1	56.6	57	20.2	24.9	20.4	25.1	19.0	23.4
							58	19.5	24.1	19.6	24.3	18.3	22.7
21	51.9	58.4	52.5	58.9	48.2	55.7	59	18.8	23.3	18.9	23.4	17.7	21.9
22	51.0	57.5	51.5	57.9	47.3	54.7	60	18.0	22.5	18.2	22.6	17.0	21.2
23	50.1	56.5	50.6	56.9	46.4	53.7							
24	49.2	55.5	49.7	56.0	45.5	52.8	61	17.3	21.7	17.5	21.8	16.4	20.5
25	48.2	54.6	48.8	55.0	44.7	51.8	62	16.7	20.9	16.8	21.0	15.8	19.8
26	47.3	53.6	47.9	54.0	43.6	50.9	63	16.0	20.1	16.1	20.2	15.3	19.1
27	46.4	52.6	47.0	53.1	42.9	49.9	64	15.3	19.4	15.4	19.5	14.7	18.4
28	45.5	51.7	46.0	52.1	42.0	49.0	65	14.7	18.6	14.8	18.7	14.1	17.7
29	44.6	50.7	45.1	51.1	41.1	48.0	66	14.1	17.9	14.1	18.0	13.6	17.1
30	43.7	49.7	44.2	50.1	40.3	47.1	67	13.4	17.1	13.5	17.2	13.1	16.4
							68	12.8	16.4	12.9	16.5	12.5	15.7
31	42.7	48.8	43.2	49.2	39.4	46.1	69	12.2	15.7	12.3	15.8	12.0	15.1
32	41.8	47.8	42.3	48.2	38.5	45.2	70	11.7	15.0	11.7	15.1	11.5	14.5
33	40.9	46.8	41.4	47.2	37.7	44.3							
34	40.0	45.9	40.5	46.3	36.8	43.3	71	11.1	14.3	11.1	14.4	11.0	13.8
35	39.1	44.9	39.5	45.3	36.0	42.4	72	10.6	13.7	10.6	13.7	10.5	13.2
36	38.2	44.0	38.6	44.3	35.1	41.5	73	10.1	13.0	10.1	13.0	10.1	12.7
37	37.3	43.0	37.7	43.4	34.3	40.6	74	9.6	12.4	9.6	12.4	9.6	12.1

| Age | All races | | Whites | | Other Races | | Age | All races | | Whites | | Other Races | |
	M	F	M	F	M	F		M	F	M	F	M	F
75	9.1	11.7	9.1	11.8	9.2	11.5	81	6.5	8.3	6.5	8.3	6.8	8.4
76	8.6	11.1	8.6	11.1	8.7	11.0	82	6.1	7.8	6.1	7.8	6.5	7.9
77	8.2	10.5	8.1	10.5	8.3	10.4	83	5.8	7.3	5.7	7.3	6.2	7.5
78	7.7	9.9	7.7	9.9	7.9	9.9	84	5.5	6.8	5.4	6.8	5.9	7.1
79	7.3	9.4	7.3	9.4	7.5	9.4	85	5.2	6.4	5.1	6.4	5.7	6.8
80	6.9	8.8	6.9	8.8	7.1	8.9							

Source: National Center for Health Statistics.

Now, using the appropriate number from the above table as a starting point, take the following quiz to adjust your answer.

1. *Family History*
   Add 1 year for each 5-year period your father lived past 70. Do the same for your mother.
   New total: _____ years
   _____ months

2. *Marital Status*
   If you're married, add 5 years. If you're over 25 and not married, deduct 1 year for every unwedded decade.
   New total: _____ years
   _____ months

3. *Where You Live*
   If you live in a small town, add 5 years. If you live in a city, subtract 2 years.
   New total: _____ years
   _____ months

4. *Economic Status*
   If you've been wealthy or poor for the greater part of your life, deduct 3 years.
   New total: _____ years
   _____ months

5. *Your Shape*
   If you're over 40, deduct 1 year for every 5 pounds over the weight you would like to be. If you're male, deduct 2 years for each inch your waist measurement exceeds your chest measurement.
   New total: _____ years
   _____ months

6. *Exercise*
   If you do moderate exercises regularly, add 3 years. If you do vigorous exercises regularly, add 5 years.
   New total: _____ years
   _____ months

7. *Disposition*
   If you're good-natured and placid, add 5 years. If you're tense and nervous, subtract 5 years.
   New total: _____ years
   _____ months

8. *Alcohol*
   If you're a heavy drinker, deduct 5 years. If you're a very heavy drinker, deduct 10 years.
   New total: _____ years
   _____ months

9. *Smoking*
   If you smoke $\frac{1}{2}$ to 1 pack a day, deduct 3 years; 1 to $1\frac{1}{2}$ packs, 5 years; $1\frac{1}{2}$ to 2 packs, 10 years. If you smoke cigars or a pipe, deduct 2 years.
   New total: _____ years
   _____ months

10. *Health and Health Habits*
    If you're frequently ill, deduct 2 years. If you have regular medical and dental checkups, add 3 years.
    FINAL TOTAL: _____ years
    _____ months

Source: Quiz items adapted from *Head-To-Toe Guide to Good Health* (Retirement Living Publishing Co., Inc., 1985), pp. 2–3.

to keep pace with young children learning a new language can readily attest. The aging process then is just that, a process in which the only constants are change and development. Furthermore, it affects us all. We may ignore it if we choose, but we cannot escape its consequences.

Second, as we have seen, people are living longer than ever before. Today it appears that the maximum potential length of life for humans is approximately 100 years, with estimates among some authorities running as high as 120 years. "If we keep making progress as we have in the past, then a baby born today can expect to live to 100," says University of Minnesota researcher James Vaupel. [8] If science ever uncovers the mystery of aging and we thus gain control over the aging process, the average length of life could increase significantly beyond 120 years. And since you may be around for a long time, you should make your long life as healthy and happy as possible. To estimate how long you are likely to live, complete the quiz entitled "Calculating Your Life Expectancy" on pages 15 and 16.

A third reason to learn more about the aging process is a demographic one. Because of current life-expectancy trends in the United States, elders are comprising an increasing percentage of our population. Knowledge of the aging process can provide you with insight into the typical hardships, delights, and general experiences that elders encounter day to day and year to year. Knowledge of what to expect will make aging less stressful.

A WELLNESS APPROACH TO AGING

The keys to a wellness approach to aging include maintaining physical fitness, observing sound nutritional practices, managing stress, and accepting self-responsibility for your well-being. Within such a framework, your goals should be as follows:

1. Adopt healthy patterns of thinking and of behavior.

2. Minimize the risks of disability or sickness in later life.

3. Reduce your chances of premature death.

4. Increase the number of years in which you can enjoy a vigorous and productive life.

By emphasizing education and preventive measures, a wellness approach can help reduce the risk of prolonged poor health

(continued on p. 20)

Meeting the Challenges of an Aging Nation

America is aging. The nation that was founded on young backs, on the strength, impetuosity, and hope of youth, is growing more mature, steadier, deeper—even, one may hope, wiser.

The Population Reference Bureau, a non-profit demographics study group in Washington, D.C., has projected that by the year 2025 Americans over age 65 will outnumber teenagers by more than two to one. According to the Census Bureau, by 2030 the median age is expected to have reached 41. By 2050, it's likely that as many as one in four Americans will be over 65. Many demographers consider these projections to be very conservative: By some estimates, the median age will eventually reach 50.

Three separate and unprecedented demographic phenomena are converging to produce the coming "Age Wave":

• *The senior boom.* Americans are living longer than ever before, and older Americans are healthier, more active, more vigorous, and more influential than any other older generation in history.

• *The birth dearth.* A decade ago, the birth rate in the United States plummeted to its lowest point ever. It has been hovering there since, and it's not likely to change. The growing population of elders is not being offset by an explosion of children.

• *The aging of the baby boom.* The leading edge of the boomer generation has now passed 40. As the boomers approach 50 and pass it, their numbers, combined with the first two demographic changes, will produce a historic shift in American life.

Our concept of marriage will change, as "till death do us part" unions generally give way to serial monogamy. In an era of longer life, some people will have marriages that last 75 years, while others will pick different mates for each major stage of life.

The child-centered nuclear family will increasingly be replaced by the "matrix" family, an adult-centered unit that spans generations and is bound together by friendship and circumstances as well as by blood and obligation.

More people will work at careers into their 70s and 80s. Many will "retire" several times during their lives—to raise a second (or third) family, enter a new business, or simply take a couple of years off to travel and enjoy themselves.

Even the physical environment will change. To fit the pace, physiology, and style of a population predominantly in the middle and later years of life, the type in books will get larger and traffic lights will change more slowly. Steps will be less steep, bathtubs less slippery, chairs more comfortable, reading lights brighter. Neighborhoods will become safer. Food might be more nutritious.

But the aging of America will affect more than just our institutions, lifestyles, and surroundings. The demographic changes that rearrange our society will also touch our innermost thoughts, hopes, and dreams. The gift of longevity will make us rethink the tempo of our lives as well as the purposes, goals, and challenges we face in each stage of life.

Indeed, the cumulative effect of all these changes might be an entirely new perspective on the possibilities of old age. A compelling philosophy has recently emerged from the European tradition of adult education that provides a simple yet visionary look at this issue. Referred to as le troisième age—"the third age"—this theory proposes that there are three "ages" of human life, each with its own focus, challenges, and opportunities.

In the first age, from birth to approximately 25 years of age, the primary tasks of life center on biological development, learning, and survival. During the early years of human existence, the average life expectancy of most people wasn't much higher than 25, so the entire thrust of society was satisfying these most basic drives.

In the second age, from about 26 to 60, the concerns of adult life focus on starting and raising a family and on productive work. The second age is filled with social activity; the lessons learned during the first age are applied to the social and professional responsibilities of the second. Until several decades ago, most people couldn't expect to live much beyond 60 and most of society revolved around the concerns of the second age.

Now, however, we are in a new era of human evolution: the third age of humanity. The concerns of the third age are twofold. First, with children grown and many of life's basic adult tasks either well under way or already accomplished, this less pressured, more reflective period allows the further development of the intellect, memory, and imagination, of emotional maturity, and of one's spiritual identity.

The third age is also a period of giving back to society the lessons, resources, and experiences accumulated over a lifetime. From this perspective, the elderly are seen not as social outcasts, but as a living bridge between yesterday, today, and tomorrow—a critical evolutionary role that no other age group can perform. According to Monsignor Charles Fahey, who serves as director of Fordham University's Third Age Center, "People in the third age should be the glue of society, not its ashes."

Of course, this is not a new idea in human history, but it's one that modern society's intense focus on youth has obscured. In other cultures and other times, the elderly have been revered for their wisdom, power, and spiritual force. In ancient China, for example, the highest achievement in Taoism was long life and the wisdom that came with the passing of years. According to writer and social historian Simone de Beauvoir, "Lao-tse's teaching sets the age of 60 as the moment at which a man may free himself from his body and become a holy being. Old age was therefore life in its very highest form."

Among the Aranda people, hunter-gatherers of the Australian forests, extreme old age brings with it a near-supernatural status: "The man whom age has already brought close to the other world is the best mediator between this and the next. It is the old people who direct the Arandas' religious life—a life that underlies the whole of their social existence."

In contemporary Japanese culture, a high value is placed on the unique opportunities for spiritual development offered by old age. According to Thomas Rohlen, an expert on Japanese culture, "What is significant in Japanese spiritualism is the promise itself, for it clearly lends meaning, integrity, and joy to many lives, especially as the nature of adult existence unfolds. It recognizes the inherent value of experience. And for all its emphasis on social responsibility, discipline, and perseverance in the middle years, it encourages these as a means to a final state of spiritual freedom, ease, and universal belonging. . . . Here is a philosophy seemingly made for adulthood—giving it stature, movement, and optimism."

Even in the United States, before modernization shifted our interest from the old to the young, the elderly were the recipients of great reverence. In the early 1840s, the Rev. Cortlandt van Rensselaer said in one of his sermons, "What a blessed influence the old exert in cherishing feelings of reverence, affection, and subordination in families; in detailing the results of experience; in importing judicious counsel in Church and State and private life."

According to Calvinist doctrine, which was profoundly influential during the early 19th century, living to a great age was taken as a sign of God's special favor. The more spiritually evolved elder was considered one of the elect, and therefore worthy of veneration. The elderly were highly honored in all social rituals and on all public occasions. As influential leader Increase Mather commented in the late 17th century, "If a man is favored with long life . . . it is God that has lengthened his days." The soul, the Puritans believed, grew throughout our lives, reaching its highest earthly perfection in old age.

A look at other eras and cultures offers a glimpse of the improvements in American life that can come with an aging population. But whether we can take advantage of this situation depends on whether our society can make the following changes:

• Uprooting ageism and gerontophobia and replacing them with a new, more positive view of aging;

• abandoning the limiting confines that come with viewing life as solely a linear progression and instead emphasizing the cyclical patterns of human existence, which is more appropriate to the shifting needs of an aging population;

• creating a new spectrum of family relationships that takes into account the sexual, companionship, and friendship needs of adults;

• improving the quality and availability of health care;

• providing products and services that will offer older men and women comfort, convenience, and pleasure;

• and achieving cooperation among Americans of all ages in creating a social system that is fair and equitable.

For us as individuals, whether an aged America turns out to be good or bad will depend on whether we can grow beyond the values and expectations of youth to discover a positive and expanded vision of who we might become in our later years.

Source: Ken Dychtwald with Joe Flower, *Utne Reader* (January/February 1990), pp. 82–86.

in older adulthood. The goal of this approach is to "instill an ethic of bodily and mental maintenance that would prevent chronic disease and allow the elderly to live long and vigorous lives until they arrive at death's doorstep." [9] Any effort to increase life expectancy must be accompanied by an effort to make those additional years healthier and more productive. To do otherwise places a staggering financial and emotional burden on families and on society at large.

Remember that aging is not an illness but a *natural* phase of life. Your objective should be to safeguard and retain your mental and physical health throughout all the stages of your life. Regardless of age, it is never too late to begin taking care of yourself. Preventive measures—to avoid sickness or injury and hospitalization, to reduce emotional stress, and to minimize social and environmental threats to your mental and physical well-being—all can help make the aging process a healthy one and ensure for you a full, productive, and enjoyable life—and a long one. 🅦

Aging and Its Physical Consequences

WE ALL AGE. Although we tend to think of aging as something bad or unusual, it is, in fact, a normal developmental process. Thus one way of defining the aging process is as "regular changes ... in mature genetically representative organisms living under representative environmental conditions." [1] The word "representative" in this definition is important, since it suggests one of the major features of aging, its variability from individual to individual and case to case. We all age in our own way and at our own rate. Aging is a complex and highly varied process. As a result, the number of years we have lived (our chronological age) is at best an approximate measure of how "old" we really are.

WHY WE AGE

Why we age is subject to debate. While there is general agreement on the effects of aging, experts disagree on its causes and have advanced a number of theories. But before we turn to these, we need first to consider some basic terminology.

One thing we know is that human beings, like other living organisms, cannot survive indefinitely. Rather, each of us has a finite life span, the period of time between birth and death during which we are "alive." The length of this interval depends on a number of conditions whose occurrence can affect our ability to survive. Among these are disease, natural disasters, and accidents, all of which can and do lead to the premature loss of life. Those concerned with aging, then, distinguish between **absolute human life span**, the maximum theoretical age beyond which no human can be expected to survive regardless of conditions, and

Absolute human life span: The maximum possible chronological age attainable by humans under ideal circumstances.

Table 2.1 The Maximum Verifiable Life Spans of Various Species

Animal	Years
Tortoise	150
[Human]	113
Asian elephant	60
Orangutan	58
Gorilla	55
Chimpanzee	50
Golden eagle	50
Whale	50
Horse	40
Grizzly bear	35
Domestic cat	30
American buffalo	26
Lion	25
Rhesus monkey	24
Dolphin	23
Dog	20
Domestic goat	20
Moose	17
Kangaroo	16
Rabbit	15
Vampire bat	13
Skunk	8
Rat	4
Mouse	$3^{1}/_{2}$
Shrew	2

Source: Roy L. Walford, *Maximum Life Span* (New York: W. W. Norton & Co., 1983), p. 11.

In comparison with other species, humans have a relatively long life span.

Mean human life span: The chronological age by which 50 percent of a given human population will have died, according to statistical projections.

mean human life span, that age by which one-half of all people born at any given time, say, 1980, actually do die. Needless to say, the mean human life span is always shorter than the absolute human life span ... at least thus far.

Absolute life spans vary from species to species. As Table 2.1 indicates, humans have a relatively long life span in comparison with most other members of the animal kingdom. The maximum verifiable life span recorded for humans is currently 113 years. Only tortoises live longer, and most animals live for much shorter lengths of time.

FIGURE 2.1
Life Expectancy for Different Historical Periods

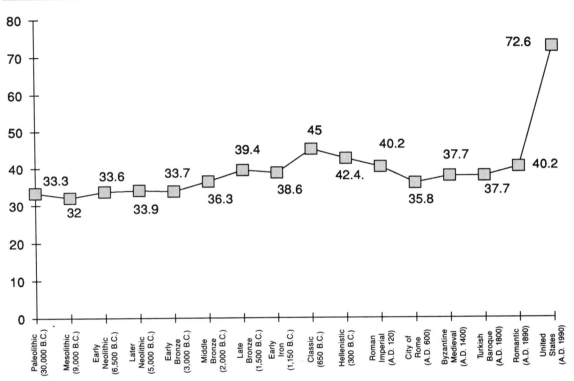

Source: Data for the United States from Department of Health and Human Services, *Health United States 1990*, p. 67; historical data from J. Lawrence Angel, "Paleoecology, Paleodemography, and Health," in *Population, Ecology and Social Evolution*, Steven Polgar, ed. (Chicago: Aldine, 1975), pp. 167–190.

Life expectancy remained relatively constant throughout history until the 20th century. Since 1900, however, it has increased dramatically in many industrialized countries. In the United States, for example, average life expectancy has almost doubled since the turn of the century.

When it comes to projecting our own life expectancy, however, mean human life span is a much more useful measure than absolute life span. While most of us might well prefer to live to 113, very few of us will. It is far more reasonable to expect that many of us will reach an age equivalent to the mean human life span. For a male born in the United States in 1988, that number is nearly 75 years. For a female born in that same year, it is over 80 years. [2]

What factors, then, do influence our life span? There are at least 4 important ones:

1. internal biological factors, primarily genetics

2. external biological forces such as disease, our overall physical condition, and chronic conditions that affect life span

3. environmental influences such as nutrition and life-style

4. social factors such as economic status, occupation, and standard of living

Together these factors interact to help determine **life expectancy**, a statistical projection of the number of years of life remaining for a specific individual or group of individuals at a particular time or place. It is important to note that life expectancy varies from individual to individual. Your life expectancy is apt to be different from that of a friend even if you both are exactly the same chronological age. Furthermore, there have been significant changes in average life expectancy over the course of human history.

One of the reasons the concept of life expectancy is so useful is precisely because it does vary from individual to individual, from group to group, and from place to place. Comparing life expectancy rates for different groups can, therefore, help us identify factors that seem to be associated with unusually long or short life expectancies. This in turn can help us devise steps to improve our life expectancy. We can do relatively little if anything about some of these factors—our genetic inheritance, for instance. But we can readily alter other factors such as our lifestyle, many aspects of our physical condition, and our nutrition. The key to healthful aging, therefore, is to identify those factors that (a) contribute to premature death or disability and (b) are controllable—and then to do something about them.

Having defined some basic terms, we can now return to the topic that began this chapter: theories of aging.

The past 2 decades have seen a dramatic increase in the amount of research on aging. One result has been a proliferation of theories of aging. While all have a certain degree of plausibility, none are totally definitive. The field is a new one, and it will be many years before researchers can sort out the competing theories and decide which are best. In the end, the theories that do survive will no doubt be the ones that view aging as the outcome of a complex set of interrelated causes rather than of any one single factor.

Life expectancy: The estimated number of years of life remaining to a given individual at a given point in his or her life span.

As we noted at the outset, there is considerable disagreement among experts on the causes of aging. Many explanations have been offered to date. These fall basically into 2 categories: theories that explain aging as the outcome of a variety of internal, biological processes—genetics, physical condition, and related factors—and theories that focus on external factors such as nutrition, life-style, and economic status. We now discuss the most plausible of the current theories.

Biological Theories

Those who believe biological factors cause aging offer 3 possible explanations. We may simply *run down*—just as a windup clock eventually winds down to a point that it stops working. Or we may *wear down*—in other words, if we were to replace the windup mechanism in a clock with one operated by a battery, the battery would eventually exhaust its capacity to run the clock and the clock would, again, stop. Finally, we may just *wear out*—in this case, the operating mechanism in the clock, regardless of whether it runs on batteries or on a windup mechanism, slows and eventually breaks down, time and use having diminished its vitality, so to speak.

All 3 of these cases involve a slowdown of biological functions, prompting scientists to ask several questions: Why does the body gradually become unable to sustain itself? Why does it cease to function? What causes the decline in its ability to produce energy? Why can't it continue to maintain the health and vigor of maturity? Why doesn't it continue to fight off harmful invasions by viruses? Researchers examining biological explanations for human aging look for answers to these and similar questions in the study of genetics, in understanding the workings of the **immune system**, and in exploring physiological control mechanisms.

Genetic Influences Several arguments support the theory that aging is caused by genetic factors. One is that different species of animals age at very different rates. But because each animal species seems to have a fixed absolute life span, there must be a biological clock at work in all living things that controls aging. Moreover, studies show that people of the same heritage share specific aging traits. For example, Caucasians tend to get gray hair at an earlier age than do Asians. [3] These observations, some believe, make it reasonable to assume that genetic information stored within each cell causes the cells to age in a predetermined way. [4] Aging, in other words, may be an outcome of preprogrammed genetic structure.

Immune system: The body's natural defense system, which works to eliminate pathogens.

FIGURE 2.2
Cell Division

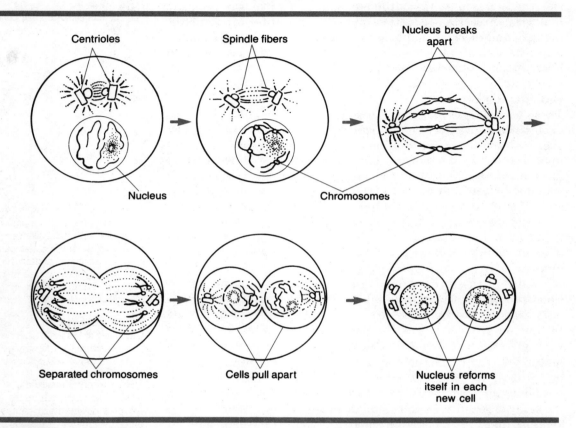

Centrioles

Spindle fibers

Nucleus breaks apart

Nucleus

Chromosomes

Separated chromosomes

Cells pull apart

Nucleus reforms itself in each new cell

The basic steps in the process by which all living cells reproduce are shown here. This process, known as *mitosis,* is essential to life, since it provides new cells for growth and replacements for worn-out cells. Some theorists believe that the aging process interferes with cells' ability to divide, thus contributing to the gradual breakdown of the body.

But advocates of a genetic explanation for aging debate *which* genetic factors affect aging, and how. For example, one theory holds that a cell can duplicate itself only so many times. According to this theory, so-called "aging genes" within each cell determine the number of rebirths the cell can experience. "Cells in the body may be biologically programmed to grow and divide only for a certain number of generations. After a predetermined number of duplications, they then lose the capacity for further growth." [5]

Others seek clues in the body's tendency to develop a hormonal imbalance over time. Doctors have tried **hormone** therapy to prevent aging in both men and women. For example, some studies have shown that administering the hormone dehydroepiandrosterone (DHEA) strengthens the immune system, lowers **serum cholesterol**, blocks the growth of induced cancer in laboratory animals, and helps control weight gain and reduce blood-sugar levels in diabetics. [6] Another group of researchers injected several male volunteers over the age of 60 with the hormone *i*nsulin-like *g*rowth *f*actor 1 (IGF-1). The scientists knew that production of IGF-1 normally declines as the body ages, which contributes to the decrease of lean body mass, the expansion of adipose-tissue mass (connective tissue in which fat is stored), and the thinning of the skin that are all associated with old age. [7] They found that the treatments helped shrink body fat, restore lean body mass, and increase the thickness of the subjects' skin. [8]

Perhaps the most widely accepted genetically based theory of aging holds that errors in **DNA (deoxyribonucleic acid)** duplication, or changes in DNA molecules, contribute to the aging process. DNA, a complex molecular structure present in every cell of all species, directs all the cell's activities, including its own perpetuation by reproduction. These molecules and the genes they contain can be damaged by radiation and heat, by chemicals such as alcohol, and by **mutation**. Mutation may occur while DNA is repairing itself or while it is producing other molecules. Researchers have also found that "self-poisons" manufactured either deliberately or accidentally in other parts of the body contribute to mutation. [9] As a result, according to researchers K. Warner Schaie and Sherry L. Willis, "damage to DNA molecules in the genetic system would result in less efficient replacement and repair of body cells, or abnormal (cancerous) cells might be manufactured instead." [10] In short, aging occurs as genetic and cellular damage accumulates, alters the cells' genetic information, and prompts further mutation.

The Immune System   Still other medical scientists support the wearing-down school of thought. They believe that the primary cause of aging lies within the body's immune system. Figure 2.3 illustrates how the normal immune system operates. Over time, however, the immune system may become less effective at recognizing and attacking deviations in the substances produced by the body. Mutated cells, which earlier in life would be attacked and destroyed by the immune system, now survive and multiply

(continued on p. 29)

Hormone: Any of the chemical substances, such as estrogen, that are released directly into the bloodstream by the endocrine glands and elicit specific responses from a targeted muscle, organ, or other bodily structure.

Serum cholesterol: Cholesterol found in the clear fluid (serum) that separates from the blood when it clots.

DNA (deoxyribonucleic acid): The extraordinarily complex double helix–shaped molecule, found in the nucleus of cells and in viruses, that stores the genetic code.

Mutation: An alteration in the structure of the DNA molecule that affects the functioning or structure of the larger organism; mutations may arise from a variety of causes, including environmental factors (radiation, exposure to chemicals) and random error during the cell division process; their effects may be either beneficial or harmful.

FIGURE 2.3
How the Body Protects Itself

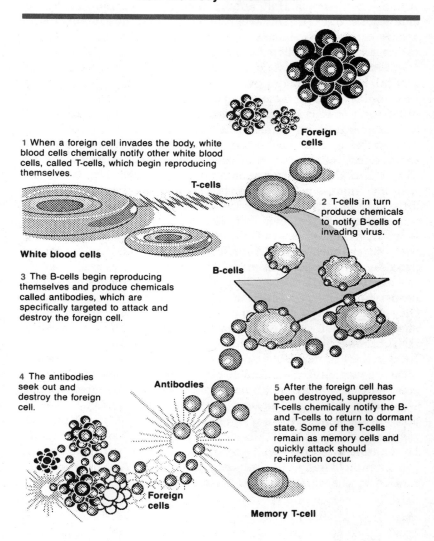

1 When a foreign cell invades the body, white blood cells chemically notify other white blood cells, called T-cells, which begin reproducing themselves.

T-cells

Foreign cells

2 T-cells in turn produce chemicals to notify B-cells of invading virus.

White blood cells

B-cells

3 The B-cells begin reproducing themselves and produce chemicals called antibodies, which are specifically targeted to attack and destroy the foreign cell.

4 The antibodies seek out and destroy the foreign cell.

Antibodies

5 After the foreign cell has been destroyed, suppressor T-cells chemically notify the B- and T-cells to return to dormant state. Some of the T-cells remain as memory cells and quickly attack should re-infection occur.

Foreign cells

Memory T-cell

Source: *Knight-Ridder Tribune News*/Terry Volpp.

The immune system is the body's defense against foreign cells, such as germs, and its means of removing its own dead, damaged cells.

in an older body. This results in a serious threat to the body as a whole, one that would not have occurred in a younger person.

A variation on this theory, the "destructive immune system responses" theory, holds that for unknown reasons, the aging body begins to err in synthesizing protein. As a result, it produces abnormal proteins. Deducing that the body has been invaded, the immune mechanism attacks the altered protein cells as it would any foreign substance. [11] An immune system particularly sensitive to mutational damage will, as a result, fail to function properly. This, in turn, makes the body more susceptible to all kinds of disease, including atherosclerosis and cancer. No longer able to recognize and eliminate damaged cells efficiently, the body begins to wear down. [12]

A third possible effect of the immune system on the aging process is the **autoimmune reaction**. When a viral or bacterial infection invades a healthy body, the immune system produces antibodies to reject or attack the unwelcome guest. The autoimmune theory holds that, with age, the immune system mistakenly produces antibodies that attack and destroy normal body cells rather than bacterial or viral invaders. [13] This theory is supported by the fact that older people suffer a higher amount of autoimmune diseases, such as arthritis, than do those under the age of 65. [14]

Physiological Controls There is a third school of thought among those who believe the causes of aging are primarily biological. This theory attributes the effects of aging to a breakdown in integrative mechanisms, not to changes in individual cells, tissues, or organs. Advocates of this theory believe that the noticeable effects of aging result from gradual deterioration in the body's ability to perform certain vital functions as it ages. [15] In other words, the body wears out.

For example, the human body tends to maintain a uniform state; it remains generally at a consistent temperature and maintains certain amounts of oxygen and sugar in the blood. Of course, the body has to work continuously to maintain these constants and does so through a process called **homeostasis**, which involves numerous organs and systems—the **endocrine glands** and the nervous system for example—all working interactively to maintain control of the body. As the body ages, the organs that produce the hormones needed to maintain homeostasis become less efficient and respond less aggressively to variations in the bodily environment. [16] As a consequence, the body becomes less able to prevent its own deterioration.

(continued on p. 32)

Autoimmune reaction: A disorder in which the immune system attacks healthy tissue or a healthy organ or group of cells that it has mistakenly identified as a harmful, foreign invader.

Homeostasis: The process by which the body regulates temperature, oxygen level, sugar content, and related factors necessary to optimum functioning in order to maintain them at constant levels.

Endocrine glands: Those glands in the body that secrete chemical substances called hormones (or endocrines) directly into the bloodstream to regulate vital bodily functions and processes; the pancreas, adrenal glands, thyroid, pituitary, ovaries, and testicles are all endocrine glands.

Winding Down

While a breakthrough drug or therapy to extend life remains a far-off fantasy, scientists are making headway tracking down clues to another mystery: *Why* do we age? What is it that builds up, goes awry or is depleted, causing the changes in physiology that we interpret as aging?

It is unlikely that these researchers will stumble on some magical potion or secret of perpetual youth, but they may make discoveries that will allow our biological functions to run more efficiently and avoid breakdowns. Their findings may slow some aging processes.

Scientists from the Soviet Union to California are testing various theories, taking care to separate what is cause and what is merely effect. Some of the so-called causes of aging put forth by researchers today may turn out to be only superficial signs of a more important mechanism tomorrow. It would be silly, for instance, to say that gray hair causes aging. Someday, when more is known about the processes of senescence, the following ideas may be as absurd.

The Tired Refrigerator Hypothesis

Scientists prefer to call this the "stochastic" theory, a more dignified name, but essentially this hypothesis holds that our bodies are like any major appliance and they wear out. (A stochastic system is a random system, one that breaks down by chance, like an old refrigerator.) This very popular theory comes in many forms and is easy for the layperson to grasp: The body is like a Volkswagen; the clutch goes, the head gasket warps and eventually it dies in a pool of oil. There's only one problem: Human beings are neither appliances nor automobiles. On the positive side, we have cells that replicate and refrigerators do not. On the negative side, sure, cars wear out, but we can intervene quite effectively to extend their maximum life spans, something we can't do with humans. The average life expectancy of an automobile is somewhere around eight years or 100,000 miles. Yet my neighbor has a '32 Ford in mint condition that runs like a top. All it takes is perfect maintenance. A 1932 Ford on the road today is equivalent to a 534-year-old human, since it has exceeded life expectancy for its species by more than seven times.

Clock of Aging Theory

A much more intriguing, and more modern, concept is that there's a genetic program somewhere in the body that dictates how fast (and in what manner) each of us will age and die. It has yet to be found, but some researchers speculate that this DNA clock might be contained in each cell, perhaps in a supergene, while others believe it resides in the brain. In fact, people have been aging and dying like clockwork for many millennia, so it's not too farfetched to believe that a hard-wired mechanism controls this genetic process.

Error Catastrophe

This theory takes many forms, but it's basically a cross between the stochastic and clock of aging concepts. The basic idea is that the genetic code that controls the production of the cells' proteins goes awry. There are two ways of looking at this: Either wear and tear damages the genetic machinery and causes these errors (the stochastic theory) or, for some reason, the "errors" are built in to the genetic code (the clock of aging theory).

The error catastrophe theory has been "pretty much demolished," according to Dr. Robert N. Butler, Brookdale professor of geriatrics at Mt. Sinai School of Medicine in New York City, as old cells now appear to do as well as young cells when it comes to protein production. It was a very useful theory for many years, however, as it spurred scientists to study the whole area of proteins and genetic error.

The Smudged Xerox Hypothesis

This one was dreamed up by the noted gerontologist Alex Comfort, better known for his book *The Joy of Sex* (Pocket Books, 1987). Think of it in this way: Take a page of *Health* magazine and photocopy it. Then photocopy your photocopy. now make a photocopy of the second photocopy, and so on. By the 50th copy, you'll have a blurry mess. Likewise with cells, says Comfort. Every time they replicate, the new copy of DNA gets more and more smudged. Comfort reportedly has since pulled away from this notion, which in fact is a variation on error catastrophe.

The Autoimmune Hypothesis

When the immune system rebels, responses may be as trivial as hay fever, as painful as rheumatoid arthritis or as deadly as lupus. In this theory, aging and death are part of one, big autoimmune disease, in which the immune system becomes confused and starts attacking the body's own cells.

Suite Genes

A person's fate depends on whole families, or "suites," of genes, say some experts. "Unless all members are perfect, you won't live as long or as well as you should," says Joan Smith-Sonneborn, who chairs the program on aging and human development at the University of Wyoming in Laramie.

Smith-Sonneborn's experiments show that there may be a way to clean up accumulated DNA damage in imperfect genes. More than 10 years ago, she made a landmark discovery in aging research when she bombarded single-cell organisms called paramecia with ultraviolet light, then shoved them under black light. The dark was known to trigger an enzyme that repaired the DNA damage caused by sunlight. What Smith-Sonneborn discovered was that these paramecia lived 50 percent longer than untreated paramecia did.

Free Radicals

It's the trendiest idea around, but in reality, the free-radical theory is simply an elegant variation on the stochastic theory. Namely, there are chemical agents called free radicals that wear down our bodies.

The Glycation Hypothesis

Another hot new theory holds that blood sugar interacts with proteins manufactured by the body's cells and distorts the genetic information. Furthering this notion is the fact that diabetics who have difficulty metabolizing sugars often contract age-related diseases such as cataracts and atherosclerosis while they are still relatively young. Edward J. Masoro of the University of Texas Health Center at San Antonio recently found that long-lived rats in dietary-restriction experiments have *low* blood glucose, thus bolstering the glycation (from the word *glucose*) hypothesis even more.

The Death Hormone

Let's finish up with a fun theory. It goes something like this: There's one part of us that lives forever—DNA, the master molecule of heredity. Human DNA doesn't want to die, so it keeps the species alive as best it can and is passed from generation to generation.

Individuals, however, are expendable. Because a species must mutate or change to keep pace with a changing environment, and because this evolution is slow, it's in that species' best interests to turn over generations as quickly as possible so that favorable mutations will show up in the gene pool.

That is the thinking behind the rather wild theory that there is a "death hormone," a substance, possibly secreted by the pituitary gland, that ages us and eventually kills us. For if we lived too long, we would hold up the process of evolution.

Source: Dick Teresi, *Health* (October 1989), pp. 56–57.

Stress: Any external stimulus, whether physical or psychological, that necessitates resistance, change, or adaptation by the individual.

Lymphocytes: The specialized white blood cells that collectively identify, attack, and destroy harmful pathogens that invade the body; lymphocytes (white blood cells) are a crucial component of the immune system.

Environment

Two external factors may play important roles in the aging process. One is the environment. Of primary concern are such factors as nutrition and life-style. Studies have demonstrated that the life spans of laboratory animals often depend on the diets they are fed. These studies have concluded that "parents would be wise to avoid overfeeding infants and children during their developmental years, especially foods loaded with fat and sugar." [17] Environmental factors, including habits and attitudes toward healthy living, are shaped early in life and owe much to the influence of parents and other significant adults.

Furthermore, a highly stressful life-style can increase our susceptibility to disease as we age. People under severe **stress** are much more vulnerable to such major chronic diseases as cancer, cardiovascular disease, diabetes, and arthritis—all illnesses that become more prevalent during later life—than those who have healthy outlets for relieving stressful daily pressures.

Finally, there are social factors to consider. Economic status, occupation, and living conditions are all potentially stressful situations. Stress triggers the release of hormones that affect both blood pressure and heart rate. Stress also lowers the level of **lymphocytes**, which are disease-fighting white blood cells, thus reducing the efficiency of the immune system. [18] Studies show, for example, that people with strong family and neighborhood support systems seem better able to recover from sickness or injury than those who lack such ties. Those who are socially isolated appear to be at higher risk of illness and premature death. Those who maintain their independence and accept responsibility for making their own choices enjoy greater health and vitality. [19]

Taken together, the various hypotheses about the causes of aging point to a combination of both internal and external factors. These factors combine and interact in a complex way. As a result, the impact of the aging process varies from person to person.

THE PHYSICAL CONSEQUENCES OF AGING

While theorists debate the primary causes of aging, no one argues about its results. We will consider only 5 of these. As we do so, however, please keep in mind 2 basic points. First, a healthy approach to living can delay the onset of the physical consequences of aging. Second, when they do occur, many of these

(continued on p. 35)

Aging and Changing: Your Body Through Time

Hair

- Thickest at age 20, our hairs shrink after that; by age 70, a person's hairs are as fine as when he [or she] was a baby.
- All people eventually turn gray. By age 50, one expert says, half of the population has a pronounced amount of gray hair.
- Twelve percent of men aged 25 are balding; 37 percent of men aged 35; 45 percent of men aged 45; and 65 percent of men aged 65.
- As a woman approaches menopause, she may get more body hair on the face, chest, or abdomen.

Brain

- Neuroscientists say that physical changes have little effect on cognitive functions. In fact, about 95 percent of all people, by most estimates, will never become senile, no matter how long they live.
- Still, almost everyone becomes slower in ability to learn and think, and memory almost always declines somewhat with age.
- Our sleep patterns change with age. According to one expert, an 80-year-old's typical pattern is 18 minutes to fall asleep, 80 percent of the night spent asleep, six hours of total sleep time, and one hour of REM [rapid eye movement, periodic movement of the eyeballs under closed lids during dream-state sleeping] sleep.

Face

- Cartilage begins to accumulate after age 30, so that by age 70, a man's nose has grown wider and longer, his earlobes have fattened, and his ears have grown a quarter-inch longer.

Height, Weight

- A woman's caloric needs drop 2 to 8 percent for each decade past age 20.

- In general, as we age, our shoulders narrow, our chest size grows and our pelvis widens. Such changes tend to occur 10 to 20 years later in women than in men. (For example, women's chest size tends to be largest from ages 55 to 64 and then starts to shrink; in men, it is largest between ages 45 and 54.)

Heart

- A person's resting heartbeat stays about the same all through life, but the heart pumps less blood with each beat. This is most pronounced during exercise, because [the] pulse can no longer rise as high as it once did.
- Although cardiovascular disease is more common in men, high blood pressure affects more women. Hypertension affects 30 percent of women in their late 50s and early 60s, compared with 28 percent of men; after 65, the sex gap widens: 36 percent of women have hypertension and 28 percent of men.

Lungs

- First, the good news: The respiratory system is one of the most resistant to change; also, the respiratory tract grows stronger with age in that after a lifetime of exposure to viruses, a person builds up immunity and catches fewer and less severe colds by middle age.
- However, a person's forced vital capacity (the amount of air that can be exhaled after a big inhalation, considered an accurate measure of vital capacity) decreases with age. Women in their 30s have an average FVC of 30 deciliters, for example, and that declines by about 3.1 deciliters every 10 years.

Abdomen

- Aging muscles in the gut tend to slacken, so it takes longer to digest a meal; cramps, gas, constipation, and a bloated feeling become

more likely. Also, with age, the stomach se-
cretes less acid, so some foods may become
harder to digest. But the lower acid also makes
heartburn less likely.

Eyesight

- Usually in the early 40s, our eyes begin having
  more trouble focusing on nearby objects and
  may need reading glasses.
- Also, as we age, our night vision weakens, we
  take longer to adjust to the dark, and we need
  more light to see clearly (by age 80, a person
  needs three times more light than at age 20 to
  see with the same clarity); our depth perception weakens; we become more sensitive to
  glare because the lens is less elastic; and,
  because our eyes' cones deteriorate, we have
  more trouble distinguishing among colors, particularly blues, greens, and purples.

Hearing

- Our hearing begins to decline in our mid-30s.
  By age 35, for example, we may have a little
  more trouble hearing high-frequency sounds
  and we may need a sound to be about 10
  decibels louder (about the level of a barely
  audible whisper) than we needed at age 25. By
  age 50, we may have trouble distinguishing
  among certain consonants—particularly *s, z,
  t, f,* and *g,* which are high-frequency sounds.

Mouth

- As we age, we get fewer surface cavities but
  more "cervical cavities," those that eat into the
  root of the tooth. Also, the gums recede.
- Also, a person's taste sensation diminishes.
- We begin to lose control over our vocal cords,
  so our voices begin to quaver. And as the vocal
  cords stiffen, our pitch rises.

Sexual Organs

- As time passes, a woman's menstrual periods
  tend to become shorter, with longer times in
  between. And women in their 30s and 40s,
  particularly those with children, tend to have
  fewer cramps.
- A woman's sexual responsiveness will reach a
  peak in her late 30s and remain on that plateau
  into her 60s (for example, women always retain
  the potential for multiple orgasm); men, however, reach their peak in the late teens and
  decline from there.
- Women's genitalia tend to decrease in size
  over the years. As a man ages, his scrotum
  hangs lower, the angle of his erections begins
  to decline in his 30s, his sperm production
  declines and the force of his ejaculations is
  less powerful.

Muscles, Bones

- The younger a person is, the more "trainable"
  his or her muscles. Aged muscles show under
  the microscope a loss and atrophy of cells,
  accumulation of fat and collagen, and loss of
  contractility. Aging muscles are less flexible
  and more susceptible to strains, pulls, and
  cramps.
- As we age, we shrink in height because the
  back muscles weaken and the discs between
  the bones in the spine deteriorate. If a man is 5
  feet 10 inches at age 30, he will likely be 5 feet
  $8^{1}/_{3}$ inches at age 70.
- A person's bones lose calcium with age, becoming more brittle and slower to heal. Joints
  become stiffer because cartilage around the
  joints is worn down and fluid around the joints
  is depleted. Also, ligaments contract and
  harden, making them more likely to tear.

Skin

- As skin ages, the oil glands that caused teen-
  age skin breakouts quit, and the skin becomes
  drier; it also thins as it loses elasticity. Because
  a man's skin is more oily and thicker, he notices
  his aging skin about 10 years later than a
  woman does.

- Skin gradually becomes less and less sensitive to temperature changes. A young woman can detect a temperature drop of 1 degree Fahrenheit; after age 65, the temperature might need to drop 9 degrees before she feels it. But skin may concurrently become more sensitive to imaginary stimuli, like itchiness.

Source: P. Insel and W. Roth, *Core Concepts in Health* 5th Edition (Mountain View, CA: Mayfield Publishing Company, 1988), pp. 514–515.

consequences can be compensated for, making it possible to continue to lead a normal life.

It is important to note that some biological changes do not result directly from aging but occur for other reasons. Biologist Bernard L. Strehler of the University of Southern California uses 4 criteria that differentiate the physical aging process from other biological processes that affect the body. Strehler maintains that a good definition of physical aging is one that acknowledges that aging is:

1. *Universal*: It should occur in all people. Just because a condition or a disease is more likely to be found in an older person does not make that condition a part of the aging process. So just because older people tend to suffer from heart disease does not make heart disease a consequence of aging. Not all older people are afflicted with it, and it occurs in younger people as well.

2. *Intrinsic*: It is a process that occurs exclusively within the person's body and is not the result of external factor(s). For example, one may find genetic damage resulting from exposure to cosmic radiation among all older people; this phenomenon is environmental, not intrinsic.

3. *Progressive*: It is a process, not an event, and the onset is both gradual and cumulative. Although a heart attack is not a characteristic of aging, the predisposing factors leading up to it may be a consequence of physical aging.

4. *Deleterious*: The effect of the phenomena or process must be negative. That such changes decrease the organism's capacity to survive is what separates them from the maturation/ growth and maturity stages in the life cycle. [20]

What, then, are some characteristic examples of physical aging? For an overview of these changes, see "Aging and Chang-

An average, sedentary man in his thirties has a vital capacity of 2 to 2.5 liters of air per minute. Thereafter, his capacity will decline at a rate of about 0.1 liters every five years to about 1.5 liters per minute at age 65 and 1 liter at age 80.

Metabolize: To transform food into energy by breaking down large molecules into smaller ones, releasing energy in the process; the general process by which the body performs this function is known as the *metabolic process* or *metabolism*.

Atherosclerosis: A narrowing of the arteries caused by the buildup of fatty deposits (plaque) on the interior walls of the arteries.

Vital capacity: The maximum volume of air that can be expelled from the lungs after inhaling to one's maximum capacity, usually expressed as a ratio (volume of air out divided by volume of air in).

ing: Your Body Through Time," on pages 33–35. Here we will consider 5 of these in detail.

ENERGY

The proper functioning of the human body depends on the workings of its various systems. These bodily functions include the circulatory system (which supplies blood from the heart to the other body organs); the respiratory system (through which oxygen is breathed in through the lungs, carbon dioxide is produced for exhalation, and the bloodstream is oxygenated to fuel the body's organs); the endocrine system (which provides essential bodily hormones); and the digestive system (which **metabolizes**, or breaks down, food into basic nutrients for the body and into waste, which is then excreted by the body). When all bodily functions are working properly, they provide the body with energy and rid it of waste.

As a person ages, the ability of his or her body to coordinate the workings of these various systems diminishes. At the same time, the ability of each system to function at peak efficiency declines. Among the results of this dual decline is a diminished capacity to supply the body with the energy it needs. [21]

In particular, the aging process slows down the workings of the circulatory and respiratory systems. It reduces both the heart rate and the volume of blood pumped by the heart. However, the overall efficiency of the heart often remains steady despite these reductions. Although the body's ability to extract oxygen from the blood may peak between ages 20 and 45 and is cut in half by age 80, recent experiments conducted by scientists at the National Institute for Aging show that, if the heart is free of disease, blood is pumped just as efficiently in a 90-year-old as in a young adult. [22] The significant cardiovascular conditions that can occur during the aging process are heart disease and stroke. Both of these chronic disorders usually result from **atherosclerosis** and high blood pressure, not from aging. A healthy life-style can reduce your risk of suffering either condition.

Additionally, people who do not smoke and who keep fit and healthy can retain the **vital capacity** of their respiratory systems through much of the aging process. And, although the volume of oxygen that the lungs can supply to the circulatory system at age 80 is only half as much as at age 40, exercise has been shown to reduce this difference. [23] Swimming, for example, can help maintain or even increase the lungs' vital capacity.

STATURE, MOBILITY, AND COORDINATION

The human body's musculoskeletal system enables us to move about and to conduct all physical activity. This musculoskeletal system is composed of bones, muscles, and joints. Each of these plays a role in a person's physical stature, mobility, and co-ordination:

- Bones: the key element in the musculoskeletal system. Their functions include giving structure to the body, serving as an anchor for muscles, and acting to preserve calcium taken in by our diets. Calcium is critical to a variety of important functions, including conducting nerve signals, maintaining a normal heartbeat, and enabling muscle contraction. From our early 20s on, the body appears to lose more calcium than it preserves. Diet and exercise can help prevent or slow the resulting loss of bone mass.
- Muscle: These are tissues, composed of long, slender cells, that protect and support the body and that produce movement when they contract. On entering one's 50s, muscle strength can begin to decline. The loss is usually minimal, about 15 percent, until the age of 70. When we reach 80, the loss may total 40 percent. [24] Note, however, that among those who perform frequent physical work or who exercise regularly, muscle strength and mass are reduced only slightly and gradually with age. [25]
- Joints: The primary function of a joint is to allow flexibility in the musculoskeletal system. Consisting of ligaments, cartilage, and other tissue, joints enable the musculoskeletal system to move about. Joints are subject to damage from 3 sources: when muscles weakened by disuse no longer provide joints with adequate support; when greater-than-normal stress or injury damages joints; and when joints become inflamed by disease, a condition commonly known as arthritis. If they are not dam-aged, joints can withstand many years of hard use with little or no evident deterioration. [26]

A decline in the strength and flexibility of bones, muscles, and joints, then, is likely to have an effect on our stature, mobility, and coordination.

Age changes our physical stature. Shrinking in height can be attributed to loss of fluid in the cartilage of the spinal column, poor posture, **scoliosis**, or **osteoporosis**. Osteoporosis occurs when the amount of minerals in a person's bones becomes so low that fractures occur without significant cause. Osteoporosis can

Scoliosis: Abnormal curvature of the spine to one side of the body; scoliosis occurs most frequently in children and adolescents, but may also affect adults.

Osteoporosis: A disturbance of bone metabolism in which the bone mass decreases and the bones become increasingly fragile.

FIGURE 2.4
Height Loss Due to Osteoporosis

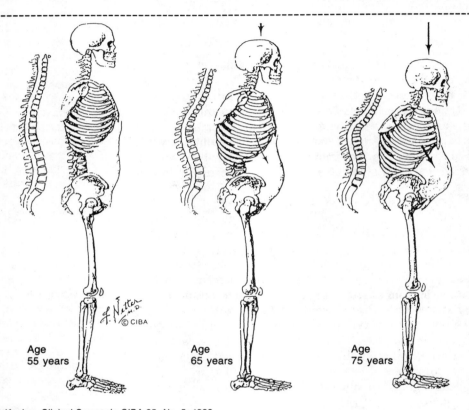

Age
55 years

Age
65 years

Age
75 years

Source: F. Kaplan, *Clinical Symposia CIBA* 35, No. 5, 1983.

Osteoporosis, a progressive loss of bone mass and strength, is an age-related condition to which women are particularly vulnerable. If left to run its natural course, osteoporosis can result in the formation of a "dowager's hump" accompanied by a significant loss of height, as depicted here. Preventive measures include increases in calcium intake and exercise.

cause a person to shrink—literally to become shorter—if his or her vertebrae are weak enough to suffer compression fractures. Other changes in our stature reflect the effects of gravity. Developing jowls, for example, or drooping eyelids or lengthened ears may be caused by the accumulating effect of gravity. Finally, older people sometimes walk with their bodies bent over, producing an exaggerated gait. According to one study, about 15

(continued on p. 42)

Osteoporosis: An Update

Historical Perspective

Osteoporosis is probably one of the few medical conditions not described by Hippocrates. So few women lived beyond the menopausal years in 500 B.C. that the effects of hormonal changes and aging on the human skeleton were not documented.

Even in the late 1800s, fragility of skeleton was considered a normal process of aging. Loss of height and rounded posture, often resulting in a humped back, [were] common among elderly Caucasian women. Who would have thought Whistler's mother might have had a disease called osteoporosis?

Discussions of fractures in weakened bones began to appear in German literature in the 1920s, and, in 1940, a Boston endocrinologist, Fuller Albright, noted that normal bone constantly breaks down and reforms and that osteoporosis might result after inadequate formation or excessive breakdown of bone.

Although little attention was paid to chronic illness during the 1940s and 1950s, these were decades of exciting developments in medicine. The era of antibiotics had arrived, advances were made in cancer diagnosis and treatment, and new surgical procedures were discovered in the arena of cardiac surgery.

In the 1960s, the heightened focus on the rights of women and the elderly increased the attention given to those afflicted with chronic illness.

Difficulties remained, though, for those women who suffered the painful effects of osteoporotic fractures. Although treatment directed toward pain relief and fracture healing was helpful, the medical profession was hampered by the lack of a diagnostic tool to measure bone mineral levels, or bone density. This prevented physicians from critically evaluating their patients' progress and it also prevented them from identifying those patients who had low bone density and were in danger of sustaining fractures.

The development of diagnostic techniques in the late 1970s, which can measure an individual's bone density, has propelled "osteoporosis" into a household name in the 1980s and 1990s.

Osteoporosis affects one in four women, and one in nine men in the United States. Approximately 1–2 per cent of the population over age 65 will sustain a hip fracture annually. The overall medical costs exceed seven billion dollars a year, but the cost in the quality of life for the individual patients [is] immeasurable. Of major concern is the high incidence of hip fractures. Because of complications that may occur following a hip fracture, there is a 30 per cent mortality rate, and only one third of patients who sustain a hip fracture will be able to resume their former way of life.

Prevention

Much progress has been made in the diagnosis and treatment of osteoporosis, but there is no doubt that acquiring and maintaining an adequate amount of bone mineral is optimal. Attempts at augmenting inadequate mineral levels, though improving, remain difficult. Therefore, it is important to identify factors that may have a negative effect on bone mineralization and those that have a positive effect. The negative factors are often referred to as risk factors.

Risk Factors

Although these are not yet fully defined, they relate to genetic, medical, and lifestyle influences on bone. These factors serve as a guideline in identifying those persons who are most likely to be at risk for developing osteoporosis.

Women are more likely to develop osteoporosis than men, as they are usually smaller in body frame and, more important, experience changes in reproductive hormone levels at least two decades before men. One in four post-menopausal women in the United States will develop osteoporosis. General risk factors include Northern European ancestry, fair hair and freckled complexion, a family history of osteoporosis, inadequate calcium intake, and a sedentary lifestyle.

Certain indicators are considered high risk factors. During young adulthood, the absence of a normal menstrual cycle for a prolonged duration (amenorrhea) is a very high risk factor. Menopause before the age of 45 without the protection of hormone replacement is a major risk factor. The presence of scoliosis, underlying medical problems such as thyroid disease, illness that curtails adequate weight-bearing exercises, and long-term use of medications such as cortisones, and aluminum-containing antacids also are considered high risk factors. A significant alcohol intake (over 2 ounces daily) and smoking are deleterious to bone. It is not always possible to reduce risk factors. However, an attempt should be made at reducing those one can.

In addition, it is critical for young men and women in their 20s and early 30s to employ strategies to ensure that optimal bone density is achieved. During these years, calcium and vitamin D intake, coupled with adequate exercise, is most important.

Diagnostic and Treatment Strategies

There are some solutions to osteoporosis, with new solutions on the way. It is now possible to measure bone mineral levels with high precision and minimal radiation exposure, using a simple scanning procedure. This has enabled us to identify those patients who may be at risk for developing osteoporosis, who should urgently consider estrogen replacement, or who need an alternative treatment plan. More important, these densitometry instruments evaluate the efficacy of the patient's individual treatment program.

Calcium

Calcium regulates several critical functions of the body, such as cardiac rhythm and blood pressure stability. Because of this, in a healthy person, the body will retain blood calcium levels within a normal range, but frequently at the expense of the bony skeleton.

In order to prevent calcium removal from bone, an adequate calcium intake is essential. Daily recommended calcium requirements range from 800 mgms [milligrams] for adult men and women, to 1,500 mgms for young adults aged 25–35 years and for post-menopausal women. Dairy products have more milligrams of calcium than other food sources. A dairy serving equals approximately 300 mgms of calcium. Eight ounces of milk or yogurt, one cup of cottage cheese or two ounces of hard cheese are some examples. There are non-dairy foods which are good sources of calcium, such as canned salmon or sardines (bones included) and calcium-fortified juices. Low-fat dairy products are encouraged, but even so, there is a concern about caloric intake. Calcium supplementation is a practical and appropriate approach in order to obtain the recommended daily allowance.

Calcium carbonate and calcium citrate are the two most frequently recommended formulas. Calcium carbonate has the highest concentration of elemental calcium, so fewer pills need to be ingested. Absorption is best in an acid environment, so the supplements should be taken just before a meal, when hydrochloric acid in the stomach is at an optimal level. Persons over seventy do not produce as much hydrochloric acid, so absorption in this situation is best after a meal.

Unfortunately, there is no FDA regulation governing the manufacture of vitamins and minerals. Some brands of calcium carbonate tablets do not disintegrate quickly enough in the stomach to ensure absorption. If a calcium carbonate tablet does not dissolve into fine powder within half an hour when covered with white vinegar, it is probably not disintegrating rapidly enough in the stomach to ensure absorption. (The acidity of vinegar is similar to [that of] hydrochloric acid.)

Calcium carbonate can cause flatulence and constipation at times. Calcium citrate is an excellent alternative. This is very well absorbed, regardless of the level of stomach acidity, and does not tend to cause either flatulence or constipation. Because it is lower in the amount of concentrated or elemental calcium, more tablets need to be ingested. Several studies have not only indicated its superiority in absorption, but the risk of kidney stone formation is markedly reduced.

Vitamin D

Vitamin D is critical to the absorption of calcium and also regulates bone metabolism. Lack of sunshine year round, the use of sunscreens, and less than one quart of milk a day, indicate that Vitamin D intake may be deficient. If supplemental Vitamin D is needed, the most practical solution is to take a multiple vitamin daily. Most provide 400 I.U.'s [International Units], which is the desired daily requirement.

Exercise

The early flights of the astronauts demonstrated that bone loss occurs rapidly in weightless conditions. Bone building and bone maintenance occur when the upright skeleton is stressed against gravity (weight-bearing or impact-loading exercise).

Activities such as brisk walking, treadmill, descending flights of stairs, dancing, or tennis are encouraged. Clinical experience leads us to believe that 3 hours a week of this type of exercise can decrease bone loss significantly and activities like square dancing 6 hours a week can actually increase bone mass, even in the elderly. These activities are not always possible for people who have physical disabilities.

The maintenance of adequate bone mass is important. However, the skeleton also needs the strength and support of various muscle groups. Stretching and general conditioning, such as swimming or yoga, in combination with weight-bearing exercise, is an important factor.

When physical limitations are present, exercise may need to be modified. It is important to discuss alternative possibilities with a healthcare professional.

Hormone Replacement Therapy

One out of four women lose[s] bone rapidly during the first seven to ten years after menopause. For these women, estrogen replacement may be a critical issue. Estrogen plays an important role in the prevention of post-menopausal bone loss.

Women who have reached post-menopausal age should have their risk factors for osteoporosis reviewed and have their bone density measured. If high risk factors are present, bone density is found to be low (or on serial bone densitometry testing, bone loss exceeds 2 per cent a year), estrogen replacement should be considered. A careful consultation with a physician should be entered into and the individual benefits versus risk of estrogen replacement be addressed.

Calcitonin

Calcitonin is a non-sex, natural hormone produced in the body that dramatically inhibits bone resorption. It has been demonstrated to be highly effective in preventing bone loss. . . . As it is a protein, it currently requires an injection, but advances utilizing a nasal form are nearing completion for release by the FDA.

New Treatment Directions

Clinical investigations currently are evaluating several new pharmaceutical agents. Bisphosphonate, most notably etidronate (also known as Didronel), appears to be more effective in decreasing the rate of spinal fracture than calcium alone. Injectable PTH [parathyroid hormone] and the active Vitamin D metabolite (1,25 $(OH)_2$VitD) [have] shown great initial promise. Sodium fluoride in high doses, although producing significant bone mass, [results in] imperfect formulation of the new bone and a consequent brittle product. All three of these agents, plus other drugs, continue to be carefully studied in established metabolic bone disease centers.

Summary

Osteoporosis is now a disorder of the decade. We understand the factors that lead to its presence and have developed accurate instruments to define its presence and course. A series of successful bone maintenance strategies have been established. Research continues in developing methods to reverse established disease.

Source: Joseph M. Lane and Theresa D. Galsworthy, *Arthritis Reporter* 2 (1991), pp. 2–3.

percent of people who are 60 years of age or older have developed a noticeable tendency to walk in this manner. [27]

Aging can further diminish mobility when connective tissue in the joints stiffens, when muscle strength declines, and when diseases such as arthritis strike. These conditions lessen bodily flexibility and diminish mobility, which make us more suscept-ible to suffering serious falls. Wary of such a danger, many older people purposely limit their physical activity. Ironically, a lack of activity *further* diminishes the efficiency of the musculoskeletal system, which, in turn, increases the likelihood of a fall. [28]

Scientists now suspect that muscular atrophy is primarily due to *disuse* and not to the aging process. If that is the case, and mounting evidence suggests that it is, exercise can help us keep active and mobile. A Tufts University study, for example, showed that 8 weeks of lifting at least 15 pounds with knee extensions increased muscle strength 160 percent and produced a 10 percent increase in muscle size among a group of 80- and 90-year-olds in nursing homes. [29]

COORDINATION

Coordination is a complex process involving a number of factors. The sequence of events involved in coordinated movement is:

1. taking in sensory information;

2. attaching meaning to the incoming information through perception;

3. selecting appropriate bodily action based on that perception;

4. transmitting instructions to the appropriate parts of the body;

5. initiating and completing the action. [30]

It is the systems supporting coordinated physical movement that sometimes fail us as we age. The body's organs of sensation and muscle groups retain the ability to perform well even in old age. However, age can cause a slowdown of specific brain functioning that can affect the proper workings of the entire musculoskeletal system. [31]

APPEARANCE

Age affects our appearance. In addition to the effects of gravity described earlier, our skin wrinkles, we develop age spots, our hair turns gray or (predominantly in males) may fall out altogether, and we acquire a midriff or hip bulge. Some of these changes are worthy of our concern.

Skin, for example, maintains its ability to protect the body well beyond the absolute life span. However, exposure to elements in the environment—especially the sun, pollution, and poor nutrition—causes skin to lose its elasticity. This, combined with natural changes to an inner layer of skin that cause the outer skin to relax and collapse slightly, results in the cracks and creases we call wrinkles. The effect of wrinkles, however, is cosmetic and not functional. [32]

The impact of age on appearance is more important for its mental consequences than for its effects on our physical health. If we hold a negative perception of aging and old age, the obvious cosmetic reminders that we ourselves are aging may cause fear and depression. These mental consequences (treated further in chapters 4 and 5) can have a serious effect.

OTHER CHANGES

Age causes a number of other physical changes. We mentioned earlier that the rate of change varies from person to person. The rate of change also varies from organ system to organ system. Here are but a few of the more significant of those changes.

During the aging process, a woman's menstrual cycle slows down and then stops altogether, a process known as **menopause**. This represents a perfectly natural life change; it does not affect life span and cannot be prevented by changes in one's life-style. It need not, however, have a negative impact on a woman's emotional health. One reference suggests, in fact, that many postmenopausal women are happier than they were during their childbearing years and enjoy sexual intimacy just as often. [33]

Another consequence of aging is a visual condition called **presbyopia**. Most people with normal vision become farsighted when they reach the age of 40; that is, they are unable to see things close up as clearly as they could when they were younger. By the age of 60, their retinas will receive only a third of the light they did when they were 20. Farsighted people are less able to

---

Did You Know That . . .

As women age, they tend to get more wrinkles than men. Men tend to have a thicker dermal layer (the layer under the surface skin), which may hold more moisture and thus help the skin to retain its elasticity for a longer time.

Menopause: The cessation of menstruation in the female, typically between the ages of 45 and 50.

Presbyopia: A condition in which the eye, as a result of normal aging, loses the elasticity necessary to focus on and clearly distinguish nearby objects; presbyopia normally first appears between ages 40 and 45 and can be remedied with reading glasses.

FIGURE 2.5
Loss of Function With Age

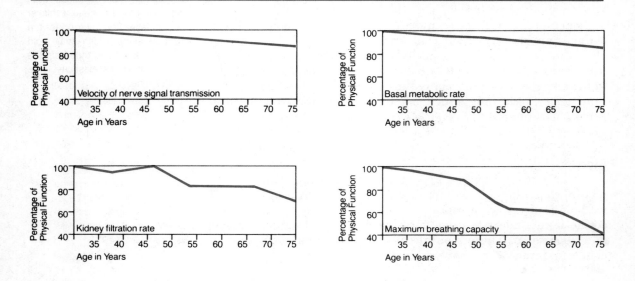

Source: Adapted from A. Leaf, "Getting Old," *Scientific American*, Vol. 229, No. 45 (1973).

The loss of function with age occurs at varying rates in different organ systems. From age 30 to 75 the basal metabolic rate decreases less than 20 percent, compared to a loss of 60 percent of a person's maximum breathing capacity.

distinguish small details and have difficulty seeing in the dark. One can compensate for most of these conditions by wearing glasses and by paying proper attention to indoor lighting.

Loss of hearing, most notably our ability to hear high-pitched tones, is yet another condition that accompanies old age. However, this change is more likely to result from abuse than aging. Studies in less industrialized, quieter societies have shown that people can hear almost as keenly when they are old as they could when they were younger. [34] Regardless of cause, hearing aids help many people compensate for hearing loss.

Older people often suffer dental problems, many of which result from the misuse, abuse, or disuse of our teeth or from chronic degenerative disease. Gums, however, do recede during the aging process, causing a higher susceptibility to cavities beneath the gum line. Periodontal disease becomes the most

(continued on p. 50)

The Mythology of Menopause

The makeshift classroom was packed with women. Though many were merely thirtysomething, they had come to hear Gail Rosselot, coordinator of health promotion at Bristol-Myers Squibb Company, talk about menopause. Scanning the room, Rosselot was intrigued by the urgency in the women's faces; more so by their youth. But the reason for the seminar's popularity soon became apparent: Many in attendance thought menopause occurred sooner than it does. Concerned about fertility, sensitive to the tickings of their biological clocks, these women were eager to understand menopause before it started.

The interest and naiveté that Rosselot witnessed is fast becoming a sign of the times. Menopause—the cessation of menstruation—is emerging as the hottest women's health topic of the decade. And for every young woman whose interest is piqued prematurely, there are countless baby boomers for whom society's sudden focus on "the change" is right on schedule. More than a dozen menopause clinics have sprung up around the country in the last few years, and pharmaceutical companies are scrambling to produce products—from vaginal moisturizers to drugs that battle osteoporosis—that cater to the postmenopausal market. These companies have the right idea. There are more than 35 million women over age 50 in this country (the average age at the onset of menopause is 51). And that number is expected to top 50 million by the year 2010, when more women will be experiencing menopause than at any other time in history.

The Double-Edged Sword

The public-health implications of the above scenario are staggering. Menopause occurs when the ovaries stop producing the female hormone estrogen. That increases a woman's risk for illnesses like osteoporosis—which causes hip and spine bones to become weak, brittle and fracture-prone—and heart disease. And more acute problems like vaginal dryness and hot flashes send thousands of women to their doctors in search of relief.

Partly in anticipation of the surging interest in menopause, the medical community is taking action. 1989 saw the inauguration of the North American Menopause Society (NAMS), aimed at furthering research on and educating health-care providers and the public about menopause. Late [in 1990], the federal government began its first major menopause study, the Postmenopausal Estrogen/Progestin Interventions Trial. Over the course of three years, the seven-center study will evaluate the effects of sex hormones like estrogen and progestin (synthetic progesterone)—used to treat several conditions associated with estrogen loss—on heart-disease risk factors in postmenopausal women.

While stepped-up research is a clear signal that doctors are taking women's health more seriously, it presents a double-edged sword. "On the one hand, it's nice to have doctors paying more attention to mid-life women," says Janine O'Leary Cobb, president of A Friend Indeed Publications Inc., in Montreal, and editor of its menopause newsletter. "Not too many years ago, any complaints women had around menopause were trivialized."

But the medicalization of this natural life process has also prompted some doctors to describe menopause as a hormone disorder. The result: Many physicians dispense hormone replacement therapy—HRT—as if it were a panacea, capable of countering the aging process and the ills that come with it. "We don't march our kids off to doctors as soon as they start menstruating. Why should we march ourselves off as soon as we stop?" asks Cobb.

According to doctors who specialize in mid-life—or climacteric—medicine, there are several good reasons. The recent flurry of research means doctors can now identify women at risk for conditions like osteoporosis and heart disease. Scientists are also developing an arsenal of treatments designed to help ease women through the peri-menopausal years (the approximately 30-year period before and after menopause).

Like Rosselot's audience, many young women regard menopause as the beginning of old age. Most middle-aged women expect it to be unpleasant, characterized by depression, hot flashes and an end to their sexual feelings. But these beliefs are bred by a lack of information. In reality, there's much you can do prior to and during "the change" to lessen potential health problems. As a result, many misconceptions long associated with menopause can be put to rest once and for all.

Myth 1: Menopause Just Happens

No, you don't just wake up one morning in a menopausal state. Up until 15 years before your period stops, you experience foreshadowing symptoms such as irregular bleeding and hot flashes—those legendary sudden bursts of warmth.

"There's a general misunderstanding that menopause lasts only one to two years, when it is really a continuum of change that occurs over several years," explains Morris Notelovitz, M.D., Ph.D., director of The Climacteric Clinic in Gainesville, Florida. Ovarian function usually begins to decline when a woman reaches her mid-30s or early 40s and is marked by a gradual reduction in estrogen levels, culminating in the cessation of monthly periods. The body begins responding immediately, in ways that can alert a woman to impending changes. Among the telltale signs:

Hot flashes. "Many women have them as early as age 38 or 40—though when a 40-year-old woman tells her doctor she has been waking up sweaty, hot flashes aren't the first thing that comes to mind," says physiologist Fredi Kronenberg, Ph.D., an assistant professor at Columbia University College of Physicians and Surgeons, who has studied hot flashes extensively. "The majority of women who have hot flashes begin them before menopause."

Menstrual irregularities. You may experience a lighter flow or a longer cycle—or skip your period altogether.

Increased PMS. Sometimes the term PMS (premenstrual syndrome) should really stand for premenopausal syndrome, says Wulf Utian, M.D., Ph.D., president of NAMS and author of *Managing Your Menopause* (Prentice Hall Press, 1990). "Most bad PMS develops in the mid-30s or later and may be related to ovarian aging," he says. Among the symptoms are cyclic recurrence of depression, irritability, mood changes, bloating and breast tenderness.

Since there's no way to know how menopause will affect you, it's wise to take stock of your lifestyle habits before it occurs. "That is the time to begin monitoring your health, exercising, eating a well-balanced diet, quitting smoking and limiting alcohol intake," says Notelovitz. "If we find in evaluating you at 35 that you have low bone mass or high cholesterol, we have another 15 years to work with you. The object is to try to get women in as good physical shape as possible prior to entering menopause. The same way that you have Lamaze during the prenatal period to ensure that you have the healthiest pregnancy possible, we're preparing you for menopause."

Myth 2: You Can't Predict When Menopause Will Occur

Menopause can hit anytime in your 40s and 50s—most commonly between ages 45 and 54. But there are clues that can help you further narrow that down.

Genetics. Family heritage plays an important role: Expect to reach menopause around the same time your mother did.

Length of Menstrual Cycle. No connection has been found between the ages at which you begin menstruation and experience menopause. But your early menstrual patterns can influence the timing of menopause. A study by Elizabeth Whelan, an epidemiologist at the National Institute of Environmental Health Sciences, found that women between 20 and 35 who had menstrual cycles of less than 26 days reached menopause an average of 2.2 years earlier than women with cycles of 33 days or more. Also, women who have regular cycles early in life tend to experience menopause earlier.

Pregnancy. Each birth seems to push the age

of menopause back a few months, so that a woman who has had five or more births reaches menopause an average of one year later than someone who has never had children.

Cigarette smoking. Smokers may experience menopause up to three years sooner than non-smokers, says Utian, director of the Cleveland Menopause Clinic. If you quit, it may come only one year earlier.

Lefthandedness. The hand you favor may also influence the start of menopause. Lynnette E. Leidy, a researcher in the department of anthropology at the State University of New York at Albany, found that the mean age at menopause among left-handed white and black women was somewhat earlier—45 years—than that for their right-handed counterparts—48.1. Among the Mexican-American women surveyed, left-handed individuals reached menopause significantly earlier—at 42.3 years versus 47.3 years for right-handed women. While further studies need to be done, Leidy theorizes that the reason may be linked to the higher percentage of auto-immune disorders in left-handed people; such illnesses could affect hormonal levels, triggering early menopause.

Myth 3: You are Destined to Get Hot Flashes

What with all the hype about hot flashes, they have become the stuff of legend—not to mention tasteless jokes. While 85 percent of women get them, experts estimate that only 10 to 15 percent have flashes severe enough to disrupt their daily lives.

A hot flash, which can occur from once an hour to once a month, is a transient feeling of warmth; however, some women become flushed, break out in perspiration, or have palpitations or dizziness. Experts aren't sure what causes these episodes. "We think the mechanism of the hot flash involves the resetting of the thermoregulatory center in the central nervous system," says Cynthia Stuenkel, M.D., director of the comprehensive menopause program at the University of California, San Diego. In other words, the hot flash seems to be the body's way of resetting its

thermostat—similar to what happens when a fever breaks.

Hot flashes become more intense as you approach menopause, and are most powerful—and common—in the first few years following it. Women who undergo surgical menopause tend to have the most severe, as their estrogen supply is cut off suddenly. The body's ability to find alternate sources of estrogen may explain why some women have more hot flashes than others, says Utian. After menopause, the ovaries continue to manufacture small amounts of androgen, a male hormone that the body can convert into estrogen. In some women, this process may result in fewer hot flashes and lower risk for osteoporosis and heart disease.

Doctors agree that currently HRT [hormone replacement therapy] is the most effective way to combat hot flashes. However, an anti-hypertensive medication called clonidine, taken orally, can minimize flashes in some women. Four hundred to 800 mg daily of vitamin E may also help.

Myth 4: You'll Lose All Desire

Probably the worst fear young women have is that menopause will signal the end of sexual feeling. While mechanical "problems" can create obstacles, there are ways to get around them.

"There are two groups of women who have sexual problems after menopause: Those who want but can't, because it hurts, and those who simply don't want," says Utian. For women in the first category (the majority), desire can fade when the loss of estrogen causes thinning of vaginal tissue and affects lubrication. "It often becomes painful to have intercourse, which may inhibit a woman's desire for sex, initiating a chain of sexual dysfunction," says Brian W. Walsh, M.D., director of the menopause unit at Brigham and Women's Hospital in Boston. Skin sensation may also diminish. "Women will say to me 'I don't feel quite the same when my husband touches me,' " Utian says.

Included in Utian's group of women who don't want sex at all are those experiencing natural menopause as well as those who have had their ovaries removed. "The latter women suffer from a loss of something, perhaps testosterone, which is normally produced in the ovaries," says Utian—and which fuels sexual desire.

Sexual problems can be handled in several ways. HRT can alleviate vaginal dryness and heighten response to touch. Very-low-dose estrogen creams, personal lubricants like K-Y jelly and vaginal moisturizers like Replens can help lubricate vaginal tissue. Some doctors prescribe desire-enhancing testosterone to women who've had their ovaries removed—though other doctors say its effects are minimal.

The best approach of all may be to "use it or lose it." "There is a natural tendency for the vagina to narrow after menopause," says Walsh. "But women who have sex on a regular basis have wider vaginas and healthier vaginal tissues."

Myth 5: Menopause Breeds Misery

Retire the notion that menopausal women turn into cranks. Researchers are finally proving what many women have long suspected: The depression and stress blamed on menopause are triggered primarily by life events, not a decline in estrogen. From coping with adolescent children to caring for aging parents and sick spouses, middle-age women can carry a lot of emotional baggage.

Menopause simply gives doctors—and unsympathetic families—an easy out, according to an ongoing study of 2,570 women begun in 1981 by Sonja M. McKinlay, Ph.D., and John B. McKinlay, Ph.D., president and vice president of the New England Research Institute in Watertown, Massachusetts. "Menopause as a physiological process provides a single, convenient, potentially treatable cause [of emotional troubles], which is attractive to a busy clinician," the McKinlays wrote. They also found that only 3 percent of the women viewed menopause negatively; others felt relieved or neutral.

[During summer 1990,] Karen A. Matthews, Ph.D., a professor of psychiatry at the University of Pittsburgh, further buttressed the growing body of evidence that menopause doesn't create mental misery. Matthews followed more than 500 women for three years; those who had recently experienced menopause were no more depressed, anxious or distressed than non-menopausal women. She also debunked the myth that menopause contributes to anger, self-consciousness, stress or nervousness.

That's not to say that the decline in estrogen doesn't have any neurological effects. Several studies have identified estrogen receptors in the brain, suggesting that estrogen is deeply involved in neurological function. And, yes, there are menopausal women who suffer from sleep disturbances and slight loss of short-term memory or ability to concentrate. But some doctors believe that these symptoms are simply triggered by middle-of-the-night hot flashes, which disrupt sleep—causing fatigue, which leads to trouble concentrating and remembering.

Myth 6: Menopause Causes Heart Disease

Not exactly. It may, however, rob women of estrogen's natural protection from it. After menopause, you're on your own and bad habits, and heredity, can catch up with you.

"Most women over 40 have at least one risk factor for heart disease—one third are smokers, 40 percent have high blood pressure and 60 percent lead sedentary lives," says Trudy Bush, Ph.D., an associate professor of epidemiology and gynecology and obstetrics at Johns Hopkins University in Baltimore. About 63 percent of women over age 50 die of heart disease.

Young women may have extra heart protection, thanks to estrogen, which keeps cholesterol levels in check and may improve circulation. (When the same women have both ovaries removed, their risk of heart disease doubles, probably because they live longer in an estrogen-free state.) But in older women who go through natural menopause, increased risk may have as much to do with unhealthy living as with declining estrogen levels.

What to do? If you smoke, stop. And don't wait until menopause to start following a low-fat diet and exercising regularly. (The American College of Sports Medicine recommends at least 20 minutes of aerobic activity three to five times a week.)

Myth 7: Once You Hit Menopause, Calcium and Exercise Won't Help Your Bones

Until recently, the word was that you had to build bone mass in your teens and 20s, by eating calcium-rich foods and participating in weight-bearing exercise. The reason: Bone density peaks and plateaus in your mid-30s; once menopause occurs, it declines by as much as 15 percent—more over time—and could put you at risk for osteoporosis.

This sage advice hasn't changed, but the end results aren't so glum. Only 25 to 30 percent of women are actually in danger of developing osteoporosis. (Most at risk are women with a family history of the disease, low body weight, a thin frame or petite stature, as well as those who abuse alcohol.)

The most exciting new research in osteoporosis indicates that calcium and exercise can help bones *after* menopause. The USDA Human Nutrition Research Center on Aging at Tufts University recently found that postmenopausal women who have low-calcium diets can reduce bone loss by bringing their calcium intakes up to RDA levels. That means 800 mg—or three servings daily—of calcium-rich foods like milk, calcium-fortified juice or green leafy vegetables. Some experts even advise women to follow NIH [National Institutes of Health] guidelines of at least 1,000 mg of calcium per day. (Calcium taken with food is more readily absorbed by the body.) And a study just out revealed that post-menopausal women with osteoporosis who took high doses of activated vitamin D prevented bone loss and increased their spine density by almost 2 percent.

There's promising news on the exercise front, as well. Women who work out regularly and vigorously have a bone density that is 10 percent higher than that of sedentary women. But while inactive menopausal women can't catch up with their more active sisters, it's never too late to save some bone. A study at Ohio State University in Columbus showed that older women who participated in a weight training program three times a week over nine months maintained their bone mineral content. Those who did no exercise experienced the normal postmenopausal decrease.

The best medicine, however, is prevention. "If you have had good nutrition with a high calcium intake and have led an active life," says Robert P. Heaney, M.D., a professor of medicine at Creighton University in Omaha, "you could easily tolerate an initial 15-percent bone loss without sustaining skeletal damage."

Myth 8: You Can't Get Pregnant After Menopause

Time was, when a women went through "the change" she lost her ability to conceive naturally. That is still a fact. But a recent study in which a group of postmenopausal women bore babies has generated a lot of interest. Doctors at the University of Southern California (USC) in Los Angeles used a variation of in vitro fertilization to implant donor eggs in five women aged 40 to 44 who had experienced early menopause. All delivered healthy babies.

While news of the procedure has prompted more than 1,000 women in their 40s and 50s to contact the researcher, it isn't for everyone. Nor is it likely to rewrite the chapter on the birds and the bees. It *will,* however, give women who've experienced premature menopause a chance at a different ending. "Up to 10 percent of women in their 40s, many of whom are reproductively active, go through early menopause. It's tragic for these women when they haven't yet had families," says Mark V. Sauer, M.D., assistant professor of obstetrics and gynecology at the USC Medical Center, who headed the study.

According to Sauer, conventional wisdom blames the high rate of miscarriages in women over 40 on aging eggs and an aging uterus. He claims his study illustrates that, with proper hormonal treatment, the uterus of an older woman is capable of maintaining a pregnancy with donor eggs. Still, many doctors say the technology is best reserved for younger women who have gone through premature menopause, in part because the older woman is at greater risk for many pregnancy-related complications.

"Older patients can have problems with gestational diabetes, hypertension, intrauterine growth retardation, hemorrhage risk, premature labor and other abnormalities," says Anne Colston Wentz, M.D., president of the Society for Assisted Reproductive Technologies and professor of obstetrics and gynecology at Northwestern University School of Medicine. But for women who were once told they were infertile or too old for conventional in vitro fertilization, Sauer remains cautiously optimistic.

Source: Lori Miller Kase, *Health* (March 1991), pp. 81–83, 85, 95.

frequent dental problem for mature and aging adults. Regular dental care can prevent or treat both conditions.

There is, then, some decline in the peak functioning of our bodily systems. But, regardless of the nature and degree of that decline, it is rarely disabling in and of itself. The harmful or fatal physical conditions that we most often associate with old age—failures of the circulatory, respiratory, digestive, or musculoskeletal systems—are a consequence of disease and not of aging. **W**

Aging and Physical Health

AGING ITSELF is not a disease. But it does have specific physical consequences. As we discussed in chapter 2, the aging body's systems sometimes slow down, weakening the body's ability to fight off disease. As a result, older people are more susceptible than their younger counterparts to a variety of acute and chronic conditions, whose effects can be a temporary nuisance or potentially fatal.

ACUTE AND CHRONIC DISEASES

Medical practitioners speak of 2 types of disorders that adversely affect our physical or mental well-being: those that are acute and those that are chronic. [1] Some people are particularly susceptible to certain disorders. Personal health habits, family history or heredity, and genetics play a decisive role in predisposing a person to a particular disease. For example, whereas one person may eat 2 eggs a day every day for 70 years without affecting his or her **cholesterol** level in a harmful way, another may have to eliminate eggs and other high-cholesterol foods altogether from his or her diet at an early age because of elevated cholesterol levels.

It is difficult, therefore, to draw many general conclusions about old age and physical health. Different individuals age in different ways and are susceptible to different disorders. If you follow healthy practices, you can often delay the occurrence of those disorders that are particularly prevalent among the elderly and lessen their impact when they do occur.

Cholesterol: A fatlike substance found in animal foods and also manufactured by the body. Cholesterol is essential to nerve and brain cell function and to the synthesis of sex hormones, and is also a component of bile acids used to aid fat digestion. It is also a part of plaques that accumulate on artery walls in atherosclerosis.

(continued on p. 53)

FIGURE 3.1
Changing Causes of Death

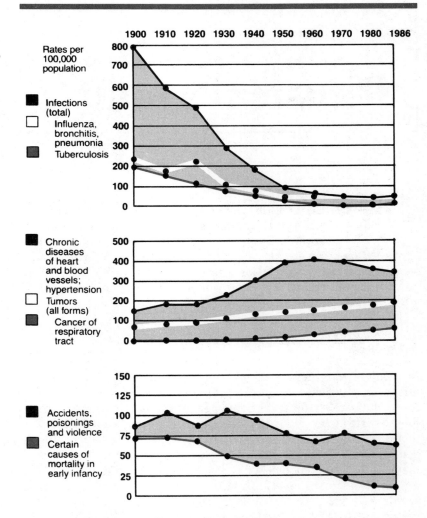

Source: Department of Health and Human Services, *Aging America: Trends and Projections* (Washington: Government Printing Office, 1990), p. 81.

Increases in life expectancy since 1990 have been accompanied by significant changes in the leading causes of death. Whereas in 1900 most people died from acute illnesses such as influenza, pneumonia, and other infectious diseases, the leading causes of death today are chronic disorders such as cancer and cardio-vascular disease.

FIGURE 3.2

Top 10 Chronic Conditions for Persons over 65

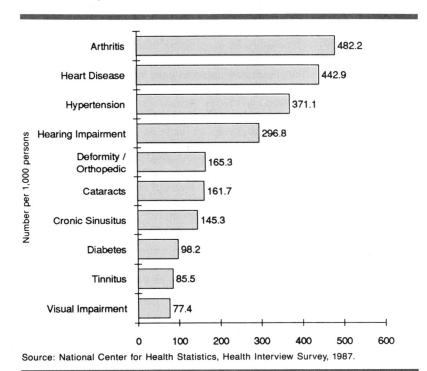

Source: National Center for Health Statistics, Health Interview Survey, 1987.

The leading chronic conditions for older adults in 1987 were arthritis, heart disease, hypertension, and hearing impairments. More than 4 out of 5 persons 65 and over have at least one chronic condition, and multiple conditions are common.

Did You Know That . . .

Four out of five older adults have at least one chronic health problem, and almost 250,000 older adults are hospitalized each year for harmful reactions to prescription or over-the-counter drugs.

Acute Diseases

A typical **acute disease** is sudden and short-term. They range in severity from such serious but easily treatable illnesses as influenza to severe, life-threatening conditions, such as pneumonia.

Studies show that the elderly actually suffer fewer acute illnesses than their younger counterparts. However, the effects of these diseases are often more serious in the elderly than in younger persons. [2]

Chronic Diseases

A **chronic disease**, on the other hand, is a long-term one, perhaps even permanent. Figure 3.2 lists the 10 chronic condi-

Acute disease: Any disease or illness whose onset is more or less sudden; acute diseases have a limited, usually brief, period of duration and vary greatly in severity.

Chronic disease: Any disease or illness that persists over an extended period of time, in contrast to acute diseases.

(continued on p. 57)

A Guide to Diseases of Older Americans

Following is a guide to the diseases of older persons that were involved in our series of surveys on "New Medicines for Older Americans."

Aging can bring with it a complex set of health problems. These diseases deprive older persons of independence by limiting their function—physically and mentally. Quality of life is affected due to pain, depression, and financial stress. Arthritis alone costs the United States $8.6 billion annually, according to the Arthritis Foundation. Great psychological and economic stress is placed on families and other caregivers. Diseases of aging deprive society of productive individuals and escalate health care costs. Some of these diseases are not well understood. In some cases, treatments are not available or have limited safety and efficacy. Often older persons must take a variety of medications to help treat their health problems, but medication to help one problem may exacerbate another. Thus there remains much to be learned about diseases of aging and the search continues for safe and effective new treatments.

ALZHEIMER'S DISEASE
Chronic deterioration of all mental functions, with average onset around age 65. It is progressive and rarely reversible. Early manifestations include decrease in attention span, impaired powers of concentration, some personality change and forgetfulness. It is difficult to diagnose, so often is not recognized at an early stage. As the disease progresses, there is loss of computational ability, word-finding problems, difficulty with ordinary activities such as dressing, cooking and balancing the checkbook, then severe memory loss and ultimately, complete disorientation, social withdrawal, and loss of independence. The personality changes may include aggressive outbursts, inappropriate sexual behavior, paranoia, and depression. The "death of the mind" has been described by both patients and family members as "the most horrible death imaginable." The increasing hours of care over many years lead to family stress, marital problems, bankruptcy, and the development of physical disorders, as well as severe depression and anxiety in the caregivers. There are no medications available that reverse the primary characteristics of the disease. Drugs are frequently used to treat symptoms, such as agitation, depression and psychosis. An estimated 4 million Americans suffer from Alzheimer's, and by the year 2040, the number of cases could be as high as 10–14 million (as published in the Nov. 10, 1989 issue of the *Journal of the American Medical Association*). More than 100,000 are estimated to have died of Alzheimer's in 1988. The Alzheimer's Association says that the cost of this disease to our society is now about $80 billion a year.

ARRHYTHMIA
Abnormal heart rhythm, usually detected by an electrocardiogram. Arrhythmias can be caused by several factors, such as coronary artery disease, heart valve problems or hyperthyroidism.

ATHEROSCLEROSIS
A common disease in which deposits of plaque containing fatty substances, such as cholesterol, are formed within the inner layers of the arteries. A common name for it is "hardening of the arteries." Atherosclerosis is a progressive condition over decades, chiefly affecting the arteries of the heart, brain, and extremities. Its complications, such as coronary artery disease and strokes, are the major causes of death in the United States.

CANCER
Cancer is second only to cardiovascular disease as the leading cause of death in older people. The single greatest risk for most cancers is increasing age. The American Cancer Society estimate[d] that more than 1 million Americans [would] be diagnosed as having cancer in 1989 and more than half of them [would] be over age 65. Cancers most prevalent among older people are: BREAST CANCER, with almost 143,000 new cases diagnosed in 1989 [killing an estimated]

43,000 women. . . . The incidence in women age 50 and older has been increasing since 1950, but the mortality rate has stabilized. COLON CANCER, [expected to] strike an estimated 107,000 persons in 1989 and prove fatal for 53,500; 94% of those diagnosed with colorectal cancer are over age 50. LEUKEMIA: ACUTE MYELOGENOUS (or MYELOID) LEUKEMIA (AML) strikes about 8,000 adults a year, with a median presentation age of 50 years and incidence increasing with age. CHRONIC LYMPHOCYTIC LEUKEMIA (CLL) strikes about 9,600 annually, with 90 percent of cases occurring after age 50. CHRONIC MYELOGENOUS (or MYELOID) LEUKEMIA (CML) strikes two out of 100,000 people in the United States each year, mainly among the middle-aged to elderly. LUNG CANCER, the leading cause of cancer deaths, whose incidence sharply increases after age 55. There [were] an estimated 155,000 new cases of lung cancer in the United States in 1989 and approximately 142,000 deaths. MOUTH CANCER, . . . diagnosed in about 31,000 people in 1989, [killing] almost 9,000. PROSTATE CANCER with an estimated 103,000 new cases and 28,500 deaths in 1989. About 80% of prostate cancers are diagnosed in men over 65. RENAL (KIDNEY) AND OTHER URINARY TRACT CANCERS, with an estimated 23,100 new cases in 1989. Renal cell carcinoma is the most common type of kidney cancer, accounting for about 75 percent of all kidney growths, usually occurring after age 40 in twice as many men as women. SKIN CANCER, including the most serious type, malignant melanoma, which occurs in about 27,000 people annually and causes 6,000 deaths.

CARDIOVASCULAR DISEASE

Cardiovascular diseases that commonly afflict older persons include arrhythmias, atherosclerosis, congestive heart failure, coronary artery disease, heart attack, high blood pressure, peripheral vascular disease and stroke. According to the American Heart Association, in 1986 almost 66 million Americans had one or more of these diseases. Heart disease is the leading cause of death in the United States, particularly among older persons, and stroke ranks third.

(See more on the individual diseases listed under their names.)

CONGESTIVE HEART FAILURE

The end result of many different types of heart disease. The heart cannot pump blood out normally. This results in congestion (water and salt retention) in the lungs, swelling in the extremities, and reduced blood flow to body tissues.

CORONARY ARTERY DISEASE

Caused by atherosclerosis of the arteries that supply the heart. Angina (decreased blood flow to the heart muscle) causes chest pain in the area of the heart. Heart attacks and congestive heart failure result from coronary artery disease. It is the most common cause of cardiovascular disability and death in the United States.

DEPRESSION

May result from a number of biologic, sociologic and psychologic factors associated with aging: decreasing mental and physical abilities, multiple medical problems, chronic pain, loss of independence, change in lifestyle such as retirement, death of friends and family members, children moving away, and economic insecurity. Early dementia and depression may be confused with one another. It is characterized by: loss of interest or pleasure in usual activities, sadness, feelings of hopelessness, irritability, poor appetite, insomnia, loss of energy, and lack of concentration. Suicidal thoughts may occur. Depression occurs in one-third of patients with Parkinson's disease and a substantial number of stroke victims. It is treatable using social support, psychotherapy and medication. About 8% of the 28.5 million people over 65 had symptoms of depression, according to 1985 estimates by the American Psychiatric Association. Many patients in nursing homes have psychiatric disorders, including depression, according to the association.

DIABETES

A chronic disease characterized by abnormal insulin secretion from the pancreas, thereby causing problems in metabolizing sugar. Symptoms may include: excessive thirst, hunger, urination, and weight loss. Diet, exercise, and weight loss are often sufficient to control this disease. Insulin treatment is needed for only a minority of elderly diabetics. Oral drugs are useful in some patients. The American Diabetes Association says that nearly 3.1 million people over 65 had diabetes in 1987 and that nearly 26,000 diabetic patients over 65 were in nursing homes. About 1 million people have been diagnosed with type I diabetes, 5 million with type II, and another estimated 5 million are undiagnosed with type II. More than 80,000 deaths were estimated to have been caused by diabetes in 1987. Total cost of institutional care of diabetic patients of all ages was $7.9 billion, the association estimates.

GLAUCOMA

An eye disease associated with increased pressure within the eyeball. If untreated, it may lead to permanent and complete blindness. Its onset is insidious in older age groups. There are no symptoms in early stages. Gradual loss of peripheral vision over a period of years eventually results in tunnel vision. 1–2% of people over 40 have glaucoma; about 25% of these cases are undetected. More than 1 million people over 65 in 1987 had glaucoma, according to the National Center for Health Statistics.

GOUT

A type of arthritis characterized by an excess of uric acid in the blood. Crystals of uric acid precipitate inside the joint cavity and set off an attack. Attacks occur suddenly, frequently at night, and often are accompanied by great pain. The feet, ankles, and knees are commonly affected, particularly the big toe. Proper drug treatment can quickly terminate the attack. About 80% of cases are in men. About 1 million Americans have gout, according to 1985 data from the Arthritis Foundation.

HEART ATTACK

A blood clot in an artery obstructs blood flow and can cause a part of the heart muscle to die due to oxygen deprivation. Sudden death may occur.

HIGH BLOOD PRESSURE

More than 60 million adults in the United States have hypertension. Without treatment, it greatly increases the incidence of cardiovascular dis-

ease, stroke and kidney failure. In about 95% of the cases, there is no known cause.

OSTEOARTHRITIS

A degenerative disease in which cartilage in the joints is worn away and reactive bony deposits form. It is the most common form of joint disease. According to 1985 data from the Arthritis Foundation, an estimated 15.8 million adults in the United States suffer from it. Incidence of the disease increases with age. It usually involves large weight-bearing joints, such as those of the hip, knee and lumbar spine, and tends to occur in joints that are damaged by diseases such as rheumatoid arthritis, by trauma such as a fracture, by occupational overuse, or by neurologic disorders. Obesity may also play a role. In the late stages, joints may become deformed, motion is limited, and pain increases. It may require hip joint replacement. Spine involvement causes low back pain, which is the most common cause of loss of work among older people.

OSTEOPOROSIS

The most common metabolic bone disease in older people. It may be associated with other diseases such as rheumatoid arthritis or with the use of medication such as corticosteroids. A reduction in bone mass leads to fractures, especially of the vertebrae, hips, and wrists. One-third to one-half of post-menopausal white females suffer from it in the United States. 25% of all white females over age 70 eventually develop fractures, loss of height, or chronic back pain due to vertebral compression. Collapsed or compressed vertebrae produce "dowager's hump." Fractures can cause catastrophic deterioration in quality of life and staggering expenses. According to the National Osteoporosis Foundation, in 1987, the estimated direct and indirect costs due to osteoporosis and associated fractures were $10 billion—and the costs are rising. Estrogen replacement therapy, calcium therapy, exercise, and other changes in lifestyle can play a role in prevention and treatment.

PARKINSON'S DISEASE

Chronic neurologic disease of unknown cause, characterized by tremors, rigidity and an abnormal gait. There is an imbalance in the body of dopamine and acetylcholine, neurotransmitters normally present in the brain. Drug therapies may help restore this balance, but they may also cause serious side effects. Some patients with advanced disease develop dementia. It is one of the most common chronic neurological diseases of later life. The United Parkinson's Foundation estimates that the average age of onset is early sixties; 3–5% of the population over 65 has Parkinson's. The organization estimates that about 10% of Parkinson's patients go to nursing homes. In the late stages of the disease, patients cannot wash, dress or feed themselves.

PERIPHERAL VASCULAR DISEASE
The obstruction of blood supply to the extremities, particularly the legs, caused by atherosclerosis.

RHEUMATOID ARTHRITIS
A chronic inflammatory disease of unknown cause. It chiefly affects the synovial membranes—thin linings—of the joints, primarily the small joints of the hands, wrists, and feet, but also can involve larger joints—the knees, ankles, and cervical spine. Symptoms include morning stiffness, joint swelling, and pain. Can eventually cause joint deformities. Incidence and prevalence of this disease increases with age. Female patients outnumber males almost 3:1. Rheumatoid arthritis peaks in males of age 60–69 and in females 50–59. More than 2 million people have rheumatoid arthritis, according to 1985 data from the Arthritis Foundation.

STROKE
Usually caused by atherosclerosis. A blood clot obstructs a major blood vessel of the brain. It results in death or serious brain damage, such as paralysis or loss of speech.

Source: "New Medicines for Older Americans," Pharmaceutical Manufacturers Association, 1989.

tions that most frequently affect those over 65 years of age. In general, the incidence of these diseases increases with age. Most older persons eventually experience at least one chronic condition. [3] Moreover, according to recent statistics, the single largest group among those who are admitted to hospitals or who visit private doctors' offices are older people with chronic diseases. [4]

SLOWING OR LIMITING THE PHYSICAL EFFECTS OF AGING

Old age invariably ends with death. But death need not, and should not, occur prematurely. Nor does it need to be accompanied by a long-term, disabling illness. Unfortunately, many people do die prematurely, "before their time," as we sometimes say. Often this is because they fail to take proper precautions to ensure their continued good health. As inhabitants of a comfortable, often sedentary, environment, Americans do not always follow sound health practices. Instead, we "sacrifice our optimal health by smoking, eat a poor diet, overeat, abuse alcohol and drugs,

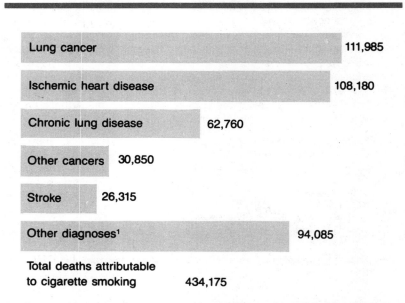

FIGURE 3.3
U.S. Deaths Attributable to Smoking, 1988

Lung cancer	111,985
Ischemic heart disease	108,180
Chronic lung disease	62,760
Other cancers	30,850
Stroke	26,315
Other diagnoses[1]	94,085

Total deaths attributable
to cigarette smoking   434,175

[1]Includes deaths from rheumatic and pulmonary heart disease, cardiac arrest, hypertension, atherosclerosis, aortic aneurysm, other arterial diseases, respiratory tuberculosis, pneumonia, influenza, low birth weight, respiratory distress syndrome, newborn respiratory conditions, sudden infant death syndrome, burn deaths, and passive smoking deaths.

Source: Office on Smoking and Health, Centers for Disease Control, Rockville, MD.

If you are a smoker, the single most useful step you can take to improve your chances of enjoying a healthy old age is to stop smoking. The American Cancer Society estimates that cigarette smoking currently accounts for approximately 20 percent of all deaths in the United States each year—over 400,000 deaths annually. Most of these deaths are premature.

bombard our ears with excessive noise, and expose our bodies to too much ultraviolet radiation from sun rays. We ... jeopardize our bodies through neglect by sitting around most of the time, encouraging our muscles and even our bones to wither and deteriorate.... We endure much abuse from the toxic chemicals in our environment." [5]

Most of the accusations in the preceding set of charges are ones over which we can exert considerable control. Changing our behavior—modifying our eating habits, increasing our physical

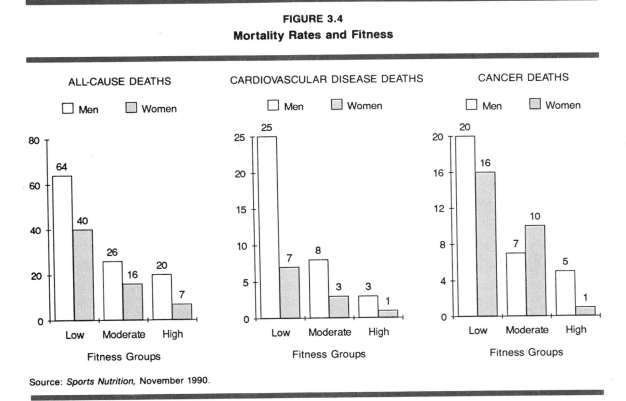

FIGURE 3.4
Mortality Rates and Fitness

Source: *Sports Nutrition*, November 1990.

According to a recent study, lack of exercise and low levels of physical fitness are significant risk factors for disease and early death. As the graphs shown here demonstrate, increases in fitness lead to a striking decline in death rates for both men and women.

activity, avoiding cigarettes, toxic chemicals, and **ultraviolet rays**, and finding healthy outlets for stress—can keep us well longer. And people who are well longer can often expect to live longer.

If you expect to live longer, if you seek to forestall the physical consequences of aging or, when they cannot be forestalled, to adjust to them, you can take one or both of 2 steps: prevention and/or compensation.

Prevention
Health and science experts are constantly studying ways to delay the aging process. Their work has uncovered some proven factors that can extend your life span:

Ultraviolet rays: Light rays whose wavelength is less than that of the shortest visible light yet longer than that of X rays; prolonged exposure to ultraviolet light is potentially harmful.

- improved nutrition
- advances in medical science
- better medical care
- advances in **pharmacology**
- fewer accidents
- improvements in sanitation
- increased attention to personal hygiene
- a healthier life-style
- greater emphasis on fitness

Pharmacology: The branch of medicine concerned with the discovery and development of drugs used in the treatment of disease.

We will return to these factors in chapter 6.

(continued on p. 62)

How to Protect Your Body From Time

"The impact of chronological aging has been overemphasized," says gerontologist John Rowe, M.D., president of Mount Sinai Medical Center in New York City. "A substantial portion of the physical changes we consider natural to aging are actually due to environmental toxins, lack of exercise, poor diet and such bad habits as smoking and excessive drinking." Based on these new findings, a growing number of researchers believe that with healthy lifestyles **we may be able to set back the biological clock—or at least slow it—by as much as forty years.**

"Almost everything we've been taught about aging is wrong," says Walter Bortz II, M.D., a physician at the Palo Alto Medical Clinic in California and author of *We Live Too Short and Die Too Long.* "We now know that a very fit body of seventy can be the same as a moderately fit body of thirty."

What's "natural" aging?

Scientists are finding that while some parts of our bodies weaken as a natural consequence of getting older, many have a remarkable potential for remaining "young" well past middle age.

• **Reproductive system** [In late 1990,] scientists made front-page headlines with the news that postmenopausal women were capable of giving birth. It had long been assumed that after a woman ceased to menstruate, her entire reproductive system shut down. But when University of Southern California researchers implanted eggs donated by younger women into the wombs of postmenopausal women, more than half carried the pregnancies to term and gave birth to perfectly healthy babies. Although the eggs of a woman in her fifties may no longer be viable, the study showed that her uterus keeps on working.

• **Heart** At the Baltimore Longitudinal Study on Aging, scientists are meticulously monitoring physiological changes that occur during the lifetimes of more than one thousand healthy volunteers. The study, which is in its thirty-third year, has so far found that an eighty-year-old healthy heart can work as well as a twenty-year-old one. According to scientists, this is not only due to the occasional stroke of genetic luck. Like an auto engine's, the human heart's performance over a lifetime is a direct result of how well it's been cared for. A low-fat diet, regular aerobic exercise, avoiding cigarette-smoking and keeping stress to a manageable level are investments that pay off in the form of a healthy heart for life.

• **Muscles** By adolescence, we're equipped with all the muscle cells we will ever have. When we build muscle, we enlarge these cells. When we lose muscle, our cells shrink—but they retain forever the capacity to enlarge. By age seventy, most of us have lost about 25 percent of our youthful body muscle, primarily due to atrophy. As we age, we tend to become more sedentary, with exercise taking a backseat to work and family demands. But research at Tufts University's USDA Human Nutrition Research Center on Aging in Boston is reversing the assumption that major declines in muscle are part of aging.

In the study, ten frail men and women as old as ninety-six regularly worked out with free weights. By the end of the study two months later, participants had already boosted thigh muscle strength by an average of 174 percent and muscle mass by 9 percent. What does this mean in real-life terms? Five volunteers who originally could walk only a quarter of a mile per hour doubled their walking speed. Two other volunteers who had previously needed canes to walk no longer needed them at all.

Says Tufts scientist Mim Nelson, Ph.D., "Our muscles have the ability to grow and get stronger from birth until we die." By making a lifelong habit of even minimal weight-bearing exercise and resistance training (such as walking twenty minutes a day and doing leg lifts wearing ankle weights for fifteen minutes a day two times a week), Dr. Nelson believes we can keep as much as 94 percent of our muscle mass well into old age.

• **Brain** Over the course of a lifetime the brain loses millions of cells and shrinks in overall size. However, this doesn't have to translate into a weakened *mind*. Studies have shown that people who remain mentally active in old age stay much sharper than those who gradually cease to challenge their intellects—another case of "use it or lose it."

Brain-cell loss *does* mean that messages travel more painstakingly along nerve pathways, slowing our reaction times and causing short-term memory to slip. But these changes don't usually take any significant toll until age seventy—and even then they may result in a person's answering a question more slowly but no less lucidly.

• Still, not every organ ages as gracefully, even if it's free of disease. For as-yet-unknown reasons, the **kidneys** become less efficient in their ability to filter blood and eliminate waste as early as age

thirty, regardless of how healthy they are. The vast majority of the time, this simply translates into an inconvenience

By age forty-five, our **sense of smell** is becoming less keen (a physiological explanation for why your grandmother wore too much perfume whenever she wore it). By the time we celebrate our seventieth birthday, our ability to **hear** high-frequency sounds is somewhat impaired. And **seeing** nearby objects and focusing on fine details usually becomes more difficult starting at age fifty. The good news for those who were nearsighted throughout most of their lives is that the change to farsightedness can eventually (by the sixties or seventies) have a corrective effect.

Total-body insurance: a strong immune system

For most of us, the **immune system** begins to falter at about age forty; by age sixty-five we're more susceptible to a variety of illnesses—from the common cold to cancer. But these facts may not be unalterable. Blood and skin tests that measure immune response have recently demonstrated that some people pushing one hundred still have "youthful" defense systems. Genetics certainly plays a part, but it now looks as if diet—a factor completely within our control—may also play a crucial role in how our immune system ages.

A growing number of scientists believe that prematurely weakened (but not diseased) immune systems are the result of **free radicals.** Although they are present in the body at low levels as a normal by-product of metabolism, they are also in polluted water and air, radon gas, cigarette smoke, alcohol and smoked meats. The trouble starts when the free radicals we ingest from these substances overwhelm our bodies' ability to detoxify them.

Through a process similar to the way exposure to air rusts metal, free radicals destroy healthy cells and, in doing so, depress the immune system. Fortunately, however, even when our built-in defenses are overrun, we can get help from the outside. **Antioxidants,** found naturally in fruits and vegetables rich in vitamins C and E (citrus fruits, tomatoes and dark-green leafy vegetables), help keep the harmful oxidizing effects of free radicals in check.

Researchers are also investigating the broader applications of nutrients as immune-system strengtheners. The key **immune-boosting nutrients** appear to be not only vitamins C and E but also B$_6$, and the minerals iron and zinc. At a recent meeting of the American Aging Association in New York City, Ranjit Chandra, M.D., a professor of medicine, pediatrics and immunology at the Memorial University of Newfoundland, reported that by correcting vitamin and trace-mineral deficiencies (using diet and supplements), he's been able to rejuvenate the immune system in 40 percent of healthy but malnourished elderly patients.

"The immune levels don't completely revert to those seen in young people," says Dr. Chandra, "but there is a significant improvement." Tufts University researchers have had similar positive results by giving healthy elderly people large doses of vitamin E.

It is unlikely that any single factor decides how we age. Genetics, diet, lack of exercise, stress, smoking and environment all combine to create an aging process unique to your body. The good news: With the exception of genetics, all of these factors are within *your* control.

Source: Madeline Chinnici, *Self* (April 1991), pp. 128–129.

Compensation

Research is slowly putting together a picture of the aging body at work. The image they are uncovering offers encouraging evidence that when the body cannot forestall the physical effects of aging, it can compensate for some of these consequences. As it ages, the human body continuously adapts to the changes it undergoes over time. Rather than simply deteriorating year by year in an accelerating downward spiral until it wears out, the body reorganizes itself in an attempt to preserve its ability to function for as long as possible. [6] These adaptations can take 3 forms.

First, bodily systems can, either individually or in conjunction with other systems, compensate for reductions in their efficiency levels or overall capacity. The circulatory system, for instance, can adjust to and even compensate for a reduction in the volume of blood pumped to the heart, which occurs when the heart rate slows down as a result of aging. [7] Or for a more complex example involving 2 major systems, there is the ability of the musculoskeletal system to adapt itself to help compensate for reduced respiratory capacity. The primary change involved here is the loss of muscle tissue that accompanies aging. The result is a lower demand for oxygen, which compensates for the fact that our respiratory capacity also diminishes as we age.

(continued on p. 64)

Promising new therapies, surgical procedures and devices under development in laboratories across the country may soon help doctors retard or reverse many of the most painful and debilitating side effects of aging.

MEMORY MENDERS Age-related diseases like stroke can impair memory; in addition, over two million people suffer from Alzheimer's, which impairs thinking skills, behavior. Experimental research shows that memory improves when aging animals are injected with nerve growth factor (NGF), a protein-building compound naturally present in the areas of the brain that control memory. One day NGF may be used to repair brain cells damaged by Alzheimer's.

Making Better Bodies

HAIR RESTORERS One-third of women experience significant hair loss after age 30. A recent study shows that the combination of minoxidil (Rogaine) and retinoids (chemical cousins of vitamin A) will stimulate noticeable regrowth in many patients.

SIGHT SAVERS With aging, the eye's lens loses elasticity, causing farsightedness. Also, decreased blood flow to the retina may cause blurred vision. Farsightedness may one day be corrected with a new laser technique that safely reshapes the cornea. In experimental surgery, blurry vision has been corrected by implanting retinal cells from healthy donors.

EAR AIDS The aging brain becomes unable to distinguish conversation from background sounds. Older hearing aids amplified all sounds equally; but new, "smarter" devices filter out distracting background noises.

HEART HELPERS Fatty deposits narrow arteries, depriving the heart of blood and making clots more likely. Doctors have developed genetically altered cells that produce IPA, an enzyme that may trigger the clot-dissolving process when the cells are implanted in arteries. Also, a new pacemaker slows down or speeds up heartbeat to accommodate stress or exertion.

BREAST-CANCER FIGHTER One out of every 11 women will be affected by this disease. Very high doses of chemotherapy can destroy more cancer cells, but at a price: Bone marrow may temporarily stop producing infection-fighting white blood cells, leaving patients at risk for life-threatening infection. In an experimental technique, healthy bone marrow cells are removed from the patient's hip before chemotherapy and returned to the body afterward to help fight infection.

MAN-MADE ORGANS A damaged liver may have to be replaced with a donor transplant. In animals, researchers have coaxed the liver to regenerate itself. A ball of Gore-Tex (a fabric used in ski jackets)

Did You Know That . . .

Approximately 1 in 3 Americans who are 65 or older have some degree of hearing impairment.

dabbed with cells from the liver grew and functioned much like the original organ when implanted next to an ailing liver.

SPINE STRENGTHENER After menopause, bones lose density, becoming soft or brittle. A recent study showed that the drug *etidronate* can halt bone loss, prevent spinal fractures and increase bone mass.

BLADDER BUILDERS Muscles connected to the urinary tract weaken with age as collagen (a tough, fibrous protein) breaks down; incontinence may result. Surgeons are testing collagen injections to strengthen the sphincter muscle, which controls the opening and closing of the bladder. Meanwhile, the new drug *terodiline* (trade name: Micturin) is being tested nationwide; it has fewer side effects, and can be taken less often, than current drugs.

ARTHRITIS EASER Arthritis affects over 11 million women. Preliminary studies show injections of *hyaluronic acid,* a lubricant found naturally in joints and eyes, may ease movement, reduce pain. In another technique, doctors insert surgical instruments into the knee joint, smoothing jagged bone and removing irritating fragments. Doctors now computer-design artificial joints that more closely match the patient's own, allowing a more natural range of movement.

Source: Cheryl Solimini, *Family Circle* (16 October 1990), pp. 113–114.

In addition, medical science can help the body compensate for and adjust to the effects of aging. Eyeglasses can correct many visual problems. Surgery can treat cataracts and glaucoma. And many people who cannot hear as well as they once could are greatly assisted by hearing aids.

Finally, many older adults can adapt to the changes that accompany aging by making small but important behavioral adjustments. For example, some people who can no longer hear as well as they once could find that they can compensate for this loss simply by paying closer attention to the words being spoken. Those who suffer a more dramatic hearing loss can learn to read lips. Many elderly people can control and even prevent some skin wrinkling by avoiding **alkaline-based soaps**, maintaining a cooler and more humid home, and applying creams as appropriate to offset dry and wrinkled skin.

The aging process undeniably slows down bodily functions and heightens the body's vulnerability to chronic conditions and disease. Although many of the changes that the aging process brings about are inevitable, they need not be debilitating. Healthy practices, a positive attitude, and behavioral adjust-

Alkaline-based soaps: Soaps to which alkaline substances such as phosphates, carbonates, and silicates have been added in order to improve their cleaning ability in water that is acidic or contains a relatively heavy concentration of minerals (hard water).

(continued on p. 67)

FIGURE 3.5
Surgical Treatment of Cataracts

Effects of Cataract Formation   Intraocular Lens (IOL) Implantation

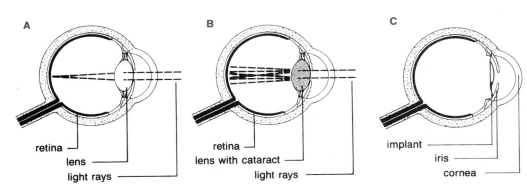

Source: *FDA Consumer,* December 1989–January 1990, p. 28.

In normal vision (A), the lens focuses light on the retina, producing clear visual images. When the lens is clouded by a cataract (B), light cannot be properly transmitted to the retina, and vision problems occur. In intraocular lens implantation, the clouded lens is removed and replaced by an implanted lens (C).

Challenge of Gravity

Fifty feet above dirt and talus, I plaster myself to a vertical wall of rock. I lift my way against the unfamiliar demands of gravity, calling on joints and muscles that suddenly seem inflexible and weak. My novice's eye can hardly make out the slender juts of stone above me that must serve as holds for hand and foot—and it requires a great leap of faith to believe in them. In the Rockies, I feel like a weak, old man. But if I fall, my brother, an expert climber, will grab me by the seat of my harness with the belay rope, and I'll hang safely, like a dangling puppet. As diapered toddlers, most of us threw our muscles and joints against the challenge of gravity with similar disregard for safety. Short, unsteady steps would lead to nosedives, sometimes broken by a belaying parental arm.

Strength, reflexes, balance and caution are physical tools we often take for granted. Falls during routine adult activities are not expected—except in the elderly. But several recent studies suggest that even in the elderly, *falls are not a natural consequence of aging.* In fact, falls are a marker for a decline in the health of the aged, a deterioration that can often be reversed.

Falls, many of which might be avoided, cause a great variety and number of problems for the elderly. Injuries are among the most common causes of death after age 65, and falls account for as many as two-thirds of these accidental deaths. Indeed, one-third of the septuagenarians living in their own homes tumble each year. Hip fractures alone lead to complications that kill one in four elderly victims. Repeated falls by a previously independent elderly person contribute to 40 percent of nursing-home admissions. Then up to 50 percent of these frail people suffer serious falls each year in the institution. With each step along this tragic course, body, mind and environment conspire to make walking, bending over to put on a shoe, or standing on a step stool as difficult as rock climbing.

The human and societal costs of falls in our aging population have led the National Institute on Aging and other government and private agencies to sponsor research on what, more precisely than we have known, contributes to falls. The focus of inquiry goes far beyond easily diagnosed medical conditions, such as an irregular heart rhythm and epilepsy, which cause falls because of sudden loss of consciousness.

The best predictors of falls in the aged, according to studies at the Sepulveda Veterans Administration Medical Center, in California, include weakness of leg muscles, problems with the body's balance system, and medications that cause fatigue, confusion or low blood pressure. These risk factors superimpose themselves on age-related bodily changes that include a decrease in muscle mass, a decline in the heart's ability to beat faster during exercise, and more resistance to movement in the connective tissues around joints and muscles. Walking itself changes with age. Our stride may shorten, the pace of our steps slows, and the time it takes to react to something in our way or to catch ourselves as we slip increases.

Stroke, Parkinson's disease and damage to the spinal cord in the neck or to the nerves that exit from the spine in the low back account for many instances of chronic leg weakness in the elderly. But the most common cause of weakness at the hips and knees and subsequent unsteadiness may arise insidiously. The overall fitness of even robust elderly people can rapidly decline after they curtail their activity when, for example, a foot becomes sore from a bunion, or joint pain flares up or an illness puts them at bed rest. Leg muscles may atrophy and joints may lose flexibility simply from disuse. Once the acute problem has been resolved and they are ready to get going again, they find themselves tiring easily, and, because of new weakness, have difficulty rising from a chair and stepping down, say off a street curb or a stair. Then, they may grow so wary of falling that they walk as little as possible, which deconditions them more and, in turn, makes them less safe in getting around their homes. The disability can be far greater if the aged person has already been slowed by a chronic disease of the heart, lung, kidneys or joints.

The downward cycle of dwindling activity and deconditioning is amplified by faltering vision and poor depth perception from cataracts or damage to the retina. It becomes more dangerous to walk, even in familiar places. Cognitive problems, such as memory loss and difficulty in planning activities or responding to new situations, can make it still less likely that the elderly person will be able to marshal the will and resources to make a comeback.

In the home, architectural barriers threaten the unwary. Poorly lighted rooms and staircases, hard-to-reach kitchen items, low toilet seats or beds that are too high or too low, slippery bathtubs and waxed floors, loose throw rugs, door thresholds and extension cords that must be hurdled, and shoes that allow skidding or that have rubber soles so thick that they catch on carpet create environmental dangers that are especially bound to trap those who are not fit.

One of the most demanding and isolating experiences for the elderly is to fall at home and not be able to get up until someone finds them. A basic principle of self-preservation—that you can get from place to place on your own two feet—and the confidence families need to have in the safety and competence of their aged parent unravels rapidly. Just one or two of those frightening moments of helplessness hasten the end to living on one's own.

How do we assess the risk for a fall? First, family members and physicians should ask the elderly mother whether or not she has fallen. A bruise, a complaint of pain or a recent change in the smoothness with which she walks may be a tip-off that she has already stumbled but has forgotten about it. Pay attention. How does she move? Physicians often do not take the time to watch their hospitalized or office patients walk. Geriatric studies suggest that we observe the elderly rising from a chair. Have the aged father stand with his eyes open and then closed, to see if he can keep his balance. Have him stand still with feet together and carefully give him a nudge on the chest, then have him turn in a circle, stand on one leg for five seconds, reach up, bend down to pick something off the floor, and sit again. If he has not been falling and can do all this without using his hands for support, and without becoming unsteady, he is probably still safe. But if he moves cautiously and awkwardly, as if traversing a wall of rock from one foothold to the next, he is not safe.

You can up the ante and have him try tandem walking, the heel-to-toe test used by the police to check for drunkenness. Those who step off a six-foot-long line several times or who grab the furniture for support are at higher risk for a fall than those who are steady. An even tougher measure of the balance mechanisms of the nervous system is to perform a few tandem steps with the eyes closed. That's like working one's

way at night from bed to bathroom with the lights out.

About half of the falls in the elderly stem from diagnosable medical conditions; about one-third arise primarily from environmental hazards; the causes of the others are unclear, even after a thorough evaluation. So prevention starts with treating potentially reversible medical problems, such as those induced by the side effects of medication, then going through a checklist of potential hazards in the home.

Still, without specific instruction and physical therapy, aged persons may not be able to increase muscle strength, improve balance, and recondition themselves to where they have built up reserves for the level of activity they want and the safety they need. Neurologic and geriatric rehabilitation programs assess and design interventions for the often subtle physical, emotional and cognitive problems that turn the elderly into timid, shuffling or, sometimes, reckless ambulators.

If we fail to identify and correct the risks for falls in the elderly who cling to the precipice, we lose the opportunity to harness our aging parents to a safety rope.

Source: Bruce Dobkin, M.D., *New York Times Magazine* (27 August 1989), pp. 36–37.

---

ments can help many elderly people adjust naturally and healthfully to the changes their bodies are undergoing. Put simply, it is often a matter of accommodating yourself to meet your changing needs. W

The Mental Consequences of Aging

I N HIS BOOK *Maximum Life Span*, Roy Walford observes that "more negative myths endure about the aging brain than all other organs combined." [1] In chapters 4 and 5, we will attempt to shed some light on the psychological issues of aging. A good way to begin this examination is for us to counter some of those myths and misunderstandings about aging, since the fears created by many of these myths can themselves contribute to the problems associated with aging. [2] To do this, we will first examine the influence of aging on the human brain and then study its effects on our sensory processes, perception, psychomotor performance, and mental functioning.

THE AGING MIND

Atrophy: A wasting away or progressive decline; degeneration.

Neurons: The impulse-conducting cells that are the basic functioning units of the nervous system.

Cerebral cortex: The outermost layer of the upper and largest portion of the brain (the cerebrum) that controls the higher cognitive functions, such as memory, speech, and thought.

Dendrites: The branching structures of a nerve cell (neuron) that receive impulses from other nearby nerve cells.

As the brain ages, its blood supply gradually declines; only half as much blood travels to the brain of a 50-year-old as to that of a 10-year-old (note that most of this reduction occurs before age 30). By age 85, a brain will have lost 10 to 20 percent of its weight, primarily a result of **atrophy**. The resulting loss of **neurons** is selective, however. Although the **cerebral cortex**, the site of higher mental functioning, will sometimes suffer a significant loss, other mental abilities remain intact; the brain matter continues to produce new **dendrites** (communication lines to other neurons) in order to compensate for any loss of brain cells. [3]

So although the brain may lose some tissue and undergo a number of changes in its neurochemical processes, this need not be interpreted as an indication of functional decline. Biologist Albert Rosenfeld observes that "the brain may simply be carry-

FIGURE 4.1
Communication Within the Brain

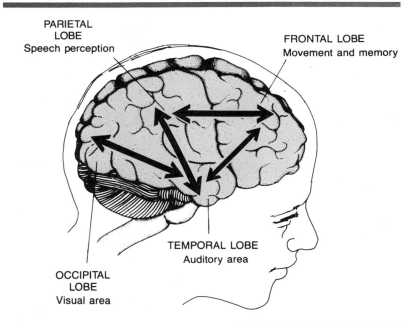

PARIETAL
LOBE
Speech perception

FRONTAL LOBE
Movement and memory

TEMPORAL LOBE
Auditory area

OCCIPITAL
LOBE
Visual area

Research now suggests that the brain's ability to perform certain complex tasks that require communication among several brain regions may decline with age. If so, this may be the result of what appears to be a general slowdown in communications between the major regions of the brain as a person ages.

ing out its work via another route, as the healthy heart seems to do. . . . Healthy people tend to retain most of their intellectual capabilities, and some even do better than ever in standard testing as they enter their seventies and eighties." [4] In sum, the loss of brain cells that results from aging is not as fearsome as it sounds. Parts of the brain continue to grow, and intelligence can increase well into one's later years. [5]

THE PSYCHOLOGICAL FUNCTIONS

The effects of aging upon many of our basic psychoneurological processes, such as our senses, perception, and psychomotor performance, are apparent and fairly easy to measure. Less clear is

(continued on p. 73)

The Aging Brain

Old age's ravages on the human body are inevitable: the eyes dim, the skin sags, the muscles soften. But the common belief that the mind too loses its edge may be just a misperception.

A new set of scientific studies suggests that the brain does not necessarily lose function or reasoning ability as it ages. Actual disease, not age in itself, may underline many or even most cases of feeblemindedness in the elderly, according to the new interpretations.

"Most notions about aging and the brain are based on folklore rather than fact," said Dr. Zaven Khachaturian, a director of research at the National Institute on Aging. "If you really study aging carefully and look at it in the absence of disease, there is no reason to believe that aging per se leads to decline and loss of cognitive and intellectual activities."

"It is clear that there's a population of old people that escapes in some sense, whose brain function is like that of a younger person," said Dr. Fred Plum of New York Hospital-Cornell Medical Center.

There is no doubt the brain does change with age. As even the most optimistic scientists readily admit, the brain shrinks as it ages, losing about 10 percent in weight, and some large nerve cells wither. The importance of these changes is hard to interpret, because so little is still understood about how the brain works. But it has been natural to interpret them as degenerative, if only because scientists as well as the general public have assumed that old people tend to be less mentally agile than younger people.

Society acknowledges the greater wisdom of older people in some contexts. Federal judges, for example, have no retirement limit imposed on them. Nor do the President or members of Congress. But in many other situations, from business to academe, the assumption is that people's mental power inevitably declines. The Fields medal, the highest honor in mathematics, is by tradition awarded to people under 40, on the assumption that they will be too old to make further important discoveries after that age.

Challenges to the accepted wisdom about the aging brain's decline have been rare, in part because of the difficulty of doing the necessary studies. The revisionist view of aging had its start decades ago in experiments that monitored people's mental abilities as they grew old. The goal was to assess which changes in mental functioning are inexorable and which are due to faltering health. Because the participants had to be followed for many years, these studies are only now beginning to bear fruit.

Another line of evidence comes from sophisticated methods of scanning the brain's activity, which show different brain patterns in younger and older people. Scientists have also conducted experiments with animals that allowed them to track physical changes that occur as the brain ages.

Many of these studies are still in progress but their general conclusions are becoming clear, says Dr. Gene Cohen, who is deputy director of the National Institute on Aging. "Increasingly," he said, "changes that were said to be aging are now thought to be due to illness."

Dr. James Fozard, who is associate director of the institute, directs the oldest and largest of the studies that follow people as they grow old. The study, he said, began in 1958, and now includes 2,000 people aged 20 to 97. Some 59 of the subjects have been tested with the same mental tasks every other year for 25 years, Dr. Fozard said. These people, now septuagenarians, are challenging researchers' notions of what they thought would be an inevitable decline.

Items on a List

Old people are only fractionally slower in tests of mental ability, and the difference may have no practical importance. In tasks like naming a familiar object presented in a picture, a 70-year-old person takes on average up to a quarter of a second longer than he did at age 30. "This could be because older people's memories are not as good," Dr. Fozard said, "or it could be because older people have more things stored in their memory, so it takes longer to search through them."

Another test is to remember a list of unrelated words. A 20-year-old can, on average, remember a 10-item list after being shown and tested on it five times. A 70-year-old will only get 35 percent of the items right after five tests, Dr. Fozard said. The difference may reflect aging, or the fact that memorizing is a skill that improves with practice. Young people just out of school may just be more used to remembering lists. And old people get better at memorizing when they practice.

Another way to study aging is to focus on the best performers in a group, rather than the group as a whole. In the aging institute's experiment, some 15 to 20 percent of the old people have no detectable changes at all in their memories or abilities to reason, said Dr. Herbert Weingartner, who studies their mental abilities.

Many of the elderly who did less well on tests of mental ability turned out to have something else wrong with them, Dr. Weingartner said, such as depression, amnesia or Alzheimer's disease.

With age, Dr. Weingartner said, "you can get exaggerated changes in memory and other cognitive functions that may be a function of pathology."

In another study at the institute, Dr. Stanley Rapoport and Dr. James Haxby are comparing the mental functions of healthy people from the age of 20 to 93. "What we generally find is that the changes we see are smaller than the changes that are usually reported," he said.

Surprising Flexibility

The changes usually reported are that intelligence declines markedly with age. In fact, intelligence tests are adjusted to account for this. As people get older, they need to get lower and lower raw scores on the test to have the same I.Q. But Dr. Haxby found that when he looked at healthy people, their raw scores stayed almost constant as they aged. He said he suspects that the populations whose intelligence tests were used in the adjustments of scores for age included old people with diseases that made their minds duller. These people's scores dragged down the averages for the older age group.

"What we find is that the changes in the raw scores between the older and younger subjects are much smaller than the changes that are usually reported," Dr. Weingartner said. Most striking, he said, the old and young people got almost exactly the same average raw scores on the tests of verbal abilities—what words mean, for example—and on general information—like how many weeks are there in a year or who wrote Hamlet.

Other investigators, looking at the physiology of aging brains, have been surprised at their flexibility. Dr. Carl Cotman of the University of California at Irvine has found that the old brain seems just as capable as the young brain at growing new connections between brain cells.

He and his colleagues found that in both old and young rats, the brain is capable of growing new connections, in a sort of repair process, after the experimenters had damaged a particular region.

"We were surprised," Dr. Cotman said. "I had actually thought the old brain would not be as capable. But it turned out we were dead wrong."

In addition, Dr. Cotman found that both the old and young rats, in growing new connections, reactivated genes that had been turned off since infancy. Before this study, he said, "we had thought the brain was in a state of dying and that the aged brain had turned from nice plastic healthy neurons into a rigid metallic type structure that was brittle and not capable of modification."

It would be unethical to attempt such studies in people, but researchers can instead look at diseases that kill specific nerve cells and examine through an autopsy whether new connections have been made to repair the nerve-cell network. One such disease is Alzheimer's, which causes a highly specific and predictable loss of nerve cells in the brain.

Dr. Cotman found that early in Alzheimer's disease, when nerve-cell death is not yet widespread, people's brains compensate by growing new connections, just like the new connections that the rats grew.

But even in healthy people there still may be some subtle changes with age, Dr. Rapoport believes. He and Dr. Barry Horwitz, a mathematician at the aging institute, began several years ago to study the brains of young and old people with positron emission tomography, or PET scans. This is a technique that measures the rate at which glucose is metabolized in each region of the brain. Avid consumption of glucose, the fuel of brain cells, indicates vigorous mental activity in that area.

Dr. Rapoport and Dr. Horwitz wondered if the degree of communication between different regions of the brain changed with age. They found less intercommunication in the brains of old people. Areas of the neocortex, for example, that control judgment, language and orientation in time and place become less well connected to each other.

Dr. Rapoport says the finding is hard to interpret but it seems that the brain of a young person is "like an army marching in step." On the same analogy, in a 50- or 60-year-old, "the army may be moving at the same rate but it is no longer moving in step." But Dr. Cotman cautioned that another interpretation is that the brain of an older person may be better able to focus its attention. It knows just where to look for the information it needs, so it does not need to waste its efforts in communicating between brain areas that are irrelevant to the particular task.

Researchers are also asking whether some people whose minds do become duller with age could keep themselves sharp by thinking more. "How do you distinguish scientifically between a cognitive decline—a matter of not oiling the machine—from what one would call an aging decline?" Dr. Plum asked.

Many people in France, said Dr. Rapoport, have already decided that the use-it-or-lose-it

hypothesis is correct. Throughout France, he said, there are mental gymnastics clinics where older people challenge their minds with puzzles and memory games.

More Faith than Science

Many investigators say that the answer is not yet in on whether using the mind can preserve it, but evidence from animal studies indicates that mental gymnastics may, in fact, help.

When animals have to negotiate a maze to survive, they grow more connections between their nerve cells. Animals that are kept in tedious surroundings or are unable to exercise their brains lose connections between brain cells. And recent studies by Dr. Chris Gall at the University of California at Irvine show that electrical activity in the brain makes animals release a hormone, nerve growth factor, that is used to keep nerve cells healthy and growing.

But, at this point, extrapolation from the animal studies to humans is more a matter of faith than science. Still, Dr. Rapoport said, "you can't lose by keeping your brain active."

The scientists studying aging add that as they delve more deeply into the myths and folklores that they as well as most others had thought were true, they are becoming more and more convinced that the task ahead of them is going to be to change the conventional wisdom about old age.

"The majority of old people do well," Dr. Cohen emphasized. "We have to recognize when we do research and when we make public policy that negative changes are simply not the norm."

Dr. Kahaturian agreed. "It is very important to change people's mindset about aging," he said. "If we don't we're going to have a terrible society."

Source: Gina Kolata, "The Aging Brain: The Mind Is Resilient, It's the Body That Fails," *New York Times*, 16 April 1991, pp. C1, C10.

how aging influences psychological processes affected by experience, such as mental functioning, drives, and emotions. [6]

Sensory Processes

Your **senses** are the faculties that enable your mind to experience the world both inside and outside your body. Our major senses are our vision, hearing, smell, taste, and touch. The **sensory threshold** describes the minimum level of stimulation that a sensing organ requires before it begins to transmit information to the brain. This threshold does undergo some alterations with time. But most of these changes can be corrected, or compensated for, through the use of various alternatives. Here is a brief review of the effects of aging on our senses:

- *Vision:* Aging eyes lose their ability to focus and to distinguish fine detail. Our ability to respond to light also diminishes. By age 60, few people have normal vision. Surgery or eyeglasses can compensate for some vision problems.
- *Hearing:* Aging lessens our ability to hear high-pitched sounds and to distinguish those frequencies adjacent to higher pitches. Older adults can compensate for these losses by focusing their attention more carefully and, sometimes, by learning to read lips, as mentioned earlier.
- *Smell:* Although scientists debate the nature, cause, and extent of a decline in the sense of smell among elders, everyone seems to agree that our sense of smell remains adequate for daily functioning. [7]
- *Taste:* Age diminishes our ability to distinguish the 4 taste qualities (sweet, salty, bitter, and sour). Scientists believe this change may be due largely to environmental factors. Smoking, wearing dentures, maintaining poor oral hygiene, eating poorly, and taking certain medications can dull the taste buds. On the other hand, proper health habits can keep the sense of taste at a high level for many years. [8]
- *Touch:* Age diminishes the elasticity of the skin, reducing its capacity to return to normal when stretched and lessening its ability to distinguish sensory signals. As a result, people over the age of 45 often become less sensitive to touch and have a higher threshold for pain. [9]

Perception

The complex process through which we comprehend what we experience is known as **perception**. Needless to say, sensory function is essential to proper perception. Age affects not only our

Senses: A living organism's physical means of detecting changes in the environment; humans have at least 10 senses, including vision, hearing, taste, smell, touch, pain, warmth, cold, equilibrium, and kinesthesis (the ability to sense the position and movement of the body and its various parts).

Sensory threshold: The minimum intensity or level of stimulation that a sensory organ must receive before it will transmit information about the stimulus to the brain.

Perception: The process by which a living organism comes to know or experience external objects and events on the basis of information reported by the sensory organs.

FIGURE 4.2
The Mechanics of Hearing

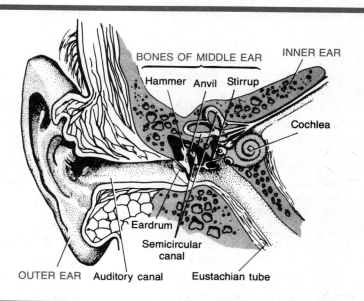

The ear is divided into 3 major components—the outer ear, middle ear, and the inner ear. The outer ear collects sound waves and transmits them to the bones of the middle ear. There they are amplified and received by the cochlea of the inner ear, which vibrates and transmits them to the temporal lobes of the brain via the auditory nerve. Hearing loss occurs when the hairs inside the cochlea begin to deteriorate, reducing their ability to detect and conduct sound waves.

ability to sense information but also the capacity of our nervous system to receive, process, and act upon that information. As a result, older people respond to many stimuli more slowly than younger people do. [10] Because of this slower response, some people become more cautious and indecisive as they age. [11]

Psychomotor Performance

Our ability to react appropriately to various stimuli is known as **psychomotor performance**. This complex process involves:

1. sensing input

2. attaching meaning to the input by perception

Psychomotor performance: The ability to react appropriately and in a timely manner to any stimulus that requires a coordinated physical (motor) and psychological response.

(continued on p. 78)

Sensory Underload

In an architecture course at the University of Michigan, students don special glasses as they tour public buildings. The effect is shocking. Well-lit corridors are suddenly veiled in twilight. Youthful gaits lose their spring and become uncertain. The students fumble for light switches that fade into the adjoining walls, and falter as they climb the stairs.

The glasses are designed to imitate the impaired vision of an elderly person. Such simulations of impaired vision, hearing and touch were developed by environmental psychologist Leon Pastalan, of the university's department of architecture and urban planning, and colleagues. Through the simulations, he tries to sensitize his students to a prevalent and widely misunderstood problem: the aging of our senses.

Signs of age develop gradually. Consequently, they often go unnoticed until the elderly person exhibits marked changes in behavior. At a crowded restaurant, a usually-spry older aunt squints, puzzled, at the menu; distracted by the background din, she ignores great chunks of dinner conversation. The scent of her perfume, usually delightful, is overwhelming now, and her subtle touch with seasonings has given way to a heavy hand with the pepper mill.

Her younger companions exchange glances and shrug helplessly. It had to happen sometime, they think. After all, she is pushing 80.

It is easy to assume that such changes are related to memory loss, confusion and other conditions often attributed to older people. Sensory losses may even be mistaken for symptoms of disease or senility, rather than normal consequences of aging, as predictable as wrinkled skin or graying hair.

Both the age when sensory losses begin and the severity of loss vary dramatically from individual to individual. Understanding how senses age can help older people—and their families and friends—fight back. Once we understand what the changes really mean, and what to expect, individuals and communities can work to minimize the negative consequences of normal deterioration of sight, hearing, taste and smell.

Loss of vision, common among older people, often occurs so gradually that it may go undetected. By about age 40, most people notice a loss of sharpness in their close-up vision. This loss occurs because the eye's crystalline lens gradually loses its youthful ability to change shape. In most cases, this problem is easily corrected by prescription lenses. In their mid 50s, most people begin to lose some ability to discriminate among colors, and eyes begin to focus at greater distances.

Other troublesome visual problems are related to changes in the pupils. In younger people, these openings in the eye respond rapidly to the changing light intensity, constricting and dilating like a camera's aperture. By age 65, the pupils have become sluggish. Also, in dim light, they no longer dilate as widely. This reduced pupil size is called senile miosis.

The retinas of someone with senile miosis receive an estimated one-third to one-tenth as much light as retinas of younger eyes. Ian Bailey, an optometrist at the University of California, Berkeley, says that at dusk or nighttime, older people see as though they are wearing very dark welder's goggles. The dimly lit aisles of movie theaters are treacherous, and reading a menu in an intimately lit restaurant may be nearly impossible. It is no surprise, then, that many are reluctant to go out at night.

Though older people cannot shed these figurative goggles, some simple steps can help. For instance, one can use a penlight to illuminate a menu or an aisle and ask a restaurateur to increase the light level.

Society can also help. If architects and public officials understand difficulties older people confront in public buildings, there are simple solutions. Light switches can be painted to contrast with walls; the horizontal treads of stairs can be covered with different materials than the vertical risers so that they can be easily distinguished.

Light levels may be increased dramatically. Careful placement of lighting fixtures is important, however, because older people are more susceptible to glare.

Hearing problems also increase with age. The high-pitched whine of a car engine, unpleasant to a young passenger, may be inaudible to the car's aged driver. Diminished sensitivity to high-frequency sounds is known as presbycusis, literally "old hearing." This problem is particularly common in industrialized societies where people are routinely exposed to high noise levels and affects men earlier and more severely than it does women. Because the condition is so common, sound-based warning systems, such as smoke alarms, must be specially engineered for older people.

Everyone experiences some difficulty understanding conversation in a crowded, noisy room, but the problem is more pronounced for older people. Many complain that they can follow conversations when there is no background noise, but that in crowds they "can't understand a thing that people are saying." Improperly designed hearing aids that amplify background noise are no help.

Of course, no one wants to appear foolish or to risk embarrassment by misunderstanding conversation or by constantly asking to have statements repeated. Consequently, some older people avoid social gatherings altogether and what began as a hearing problem leads to social isolation.

One way an older person can hear better in a crowded room is to stand in the right place, keeping these points in mind:

• The best spots for conversation are near soft, sound-absorbent materials such as drapes, bookshelves or upholstered furniture.

• Hard surfaces such as large windows or plaster walls exaggerate background noise and may create echoes.

• A high-backed chair will help shield its occupant from background clamor.

When an ideal spot for conversation is unavailable, asking people to speak more slowly may increase clarity dramatically. So can using your eyes, as Benjamin Franklin learned when he served as a special commissioner to France. In his letters, he described how difficult it was at first for him to understand conversations in French. Then Franklin discovered that when he focused on the speaker's moving lips, he was able to parse the confusing sounds into meaningful words and phrases.

Franklin's strategy can be helpful whenever speech is masked by background noise. It helps if the speaker's lips are not obscured by beard or mustache. Friends and family can help by speaking clearly and by moving their lips distinctly rather than mumbling.

Changes in taste and smell may be even more subtle than those that befall vision and hearing, but the effects are considerable: Many older people, especially the very old, lose interest in eating. In time, they may change their dietary habits and thereby become more vulnerable to weight loss, anorexia and malnutrition.

Psychologist Susan Schiffman, of Duke University Medical Center, has found that age reduces the sharpness of taste and, especially, smell. The aromas of favorite foods lose their power to entice, and the excitement of flavor yields to a bland, boring uniformity. Older people are more likely to describe the taste and smell of foods as "weak" or even nonexistent.

When Schiffman studied the thresholds at which people of different ages detect a certain smell or taste, she found that the concentration of molecules responsible for odor and taste must be 2 to 12 times more intense for a person older than 70 than for a younger person. Therefore, she says, many older people are unable to discriminate among flavors such as those associated with coffees or wines.

She asked healthy residents of a retirement home and a group of younger college students to participate in a taste and smell test. They were blindfolded and presented with a food container, which they smelled. They then were asked to taste teaspoonfuls of a variety of foods, each of which was unseasoned, steamed and blended to a soft, uniform texture. Nearly all of the foods were more accurately identified by the younger participants than by their older counterparts. For example, only 7 percent of the older participants, as opposed to 63 percent of the students, identified carrots correctly.

Schiffman also found that elderly people rate strongly flavored food as tasting significantly more pleasant than do their younger counterparts. Such age-related differences can pose a dilemma for cooks who suddenly must cater, literally, to different palates. One approach is to place seasonings on the table, thus enabling each person to season the food to taste, although older people should recognize that excess salt or sugar can be unhealthful.

Careful chewing also may help an older person experience flavors more intensely. "Swish food around more in your mouth to increase the food's contact with the tongue," Schiffman suggests. This method also will increase exposure of the food's smell to odor receptors in the upper nose. As air rises in the back of the mouth, the sensation of smell may increase. Older people, she adds, often enjoy eating roughly textured and crunchy foods. Greater variety helps compensate for the absence of strong flavors.

Several years ago, Richard L. Doty, director of the Smell and Taste Center at the University of Pennsylvania's hospital, developed a simple, inexpensive scratch-and-sniff test used to diagnose smell disorders. The test, administered by about 1,500 clinics nationwide, quantitatively measures a person's ability to smell and identify 40 odors. Test results show that 25 percent of people between the ages of 65 and 80 have major smell dysfunction and that after 80, the incidence rises to 50 percent.

Weakened sense of smell also makes it less likely that an elderly person can detect a gas leak, smoke, spoiled food or even the fumes escaping from a pump at a self-service gas station. Psychologists Joseph C. Stevens and William S. Cain of the John B. Pierce Foundation in New Haven, Connecticut, found that under laboratory conditions, older people have trouble detecting the pungent odors in substances such as ammonia. Sometimes, they found, an elderly person detected and reacted to noxious fumes only when those fumes reached levels that would be dangerous in a home or another environment. Cain and Stevens have also found that older people often cannot detect the odorant added to propane gas, a common but potentially explosive substance used to heat homes. In one of their studies, concentrations of propane were high enough to create risk of explosion before 45 percent of people over 65 smelled the gas.

In general, our sense of smell tends to remain unchanged until we reach our mid 50s, when a progressive decline sets in. Several factors may explain the decline in ability to smell, Doty said. Serious head trauma caused by falls, for example, may affect olfactory function. So may viruses, such as influenza, that attack the receptors for smell that are located in the upper reaches of the nose.

Our senses operate in a difficult environment, and the changes described here may be sobering. It is remarkable, though, that the changes are not even greater over time. The eyes you're using to read these words are the same ones you were born with, and most likely, they will bring you useful visual information for the rest of your life. For most of us, they show very little wear, even though by age 60 our eyes have been exposed to more light energy than would be unleashed by a nuclear blast. Most ears, after withstanding sound ranging from the blare of rock music to the roar of jet engines, continue to deliver high-quality information. All in all, the human senses are remarkably durable.

In some ways, it may be easier to face the prospect of changes in store for ourselves than it is to observe them in our parents and others. But it is comforting to realize that diminished senses seldom indicate a dulling of mental faculties. Not that it's fun to have dimmed vision or dampened ability to taste and smell. But good humor, compassion and inventiveness can help improve the safety of our aging parents and loved ones, so that sensory changes are bearable, if unwelcome, facts of life.

Source: Robert Sekuler and Randolph Blake, *Psychology Today* (December 1987), pp. 48–51.

3. integrating the newly perceived information with preexisting data

4. deciding whether or not action is appropriate as a response to the new information

5. signaling the affected area of the body as to the appropriate action to be taken

6. responding to the input with motor action [12]

Because aging slows down our reaction time, it often becomes more difficult to respond quickly and appropriately to a given stimulus. [13] Studies have shown, however, that many older people can compensate for this loss by concentrating solely on accuracy rather than speed. "By being more cautious and taking extra time," says psychologist A. T. Welford, "older people more than compensate for any tendency to err [as a result of] a slowed sensory-motor response time." [14] In some instances, elders have proven to have more accurate psychomotor reactions than their younger counterparts.

COGNITIVE FUNCTIONING

Cognitive functioning includes the ability to learn, remember, think, solve problems, and create. Because this higher order of thought processing is such a complex function, it is hard to say just what effect aging has on each of its elements. One important study concluded, however, that on the whole, cognitive performance remained steady until around the age of 70, then declined, but not uniformly. [15]

A review of aging's effects on the processes that comprise cognitive functioning shows the following:

• *Learning:* The ability to accumulate and apply new information and skills appears to decline with age, especially after the age of 70. The extent and importance of this decline and the reasons why it occurs are unclear. Furthermore, such a decline may have little or no impact on the quality of one's life. When it does, special training and alterations in behavioral patterns can compensate for any loss.

• *Memory:* Memory occurs in 3 stages: registration, retention, and recall. More than 25 percent of those surveyed in one study did not suffer a decline in memory function after the age of 70

Cognitive functioning: The capacity to perform the higher-order mental processes, such as perceiving, thinking, and knowing.

FIGURE 4.3
Aging and Intellectual Performance

Did You Know That . . .

The human brain is composed of cells and circuitry that share operating pathways. By one estimate, more than half of the brain's cells would have to die before any appreciable memory loss occurred.

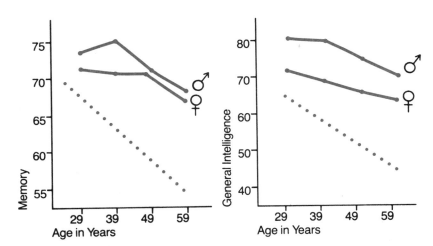

Intellectual performance in relation to age of a group of Parisian schoolteachers (——) compared to an average French population (• • • •).

Source: R. L. Walford, *Maximum Life Span* (New York: W. W. Norton and Company, 1983), p. 62.

In a study of the relationship of intellectual performance to chronological age, it was discovered that highly educated people whose work was primarily cerebral showed minimal loss of function as they aged.

and often continued to perform well on memory tests well until their 80s. [16] Overall, though, studies have shown that age lessens our ability to process information thoroughly and many therefore have trouble with recall. [17] But although memory can decline with age, this consequence may result from a lessened ability to learn rather than a failure in memory itself. Those who support this theory point to the fact that many older people have trouble with short-term memory but can perfectly remember things that happened long ago. Some studies have shown that long-term memory actually improves with age.

- *Problem Solving:* The ability to choose and use appropriate learned skills and perceptions, and to make choices from among alternatives, appears to decline with age at about the same rate as the other mental processes.

(continued on p. 83)

The Reason of Age

The golden years are making a comeback. As researchers spend less time looking at what we lose as we get older and more at what we keep or gain, aging is looking better.

Consider Andrés Segovia, still giving acclaimed concerts on the classical guitar at age 92 . . . Claude Pepper, who came in with the 20th century and has served in Congress for most of the past 50 years . . . Bob Hope, entertaining and golfing his way around the world 82 years after his birth in Eltham, England.

But aren't these people exceptions? Of course they are. Men and women with unusual abilities are always exceptions, whatever their age. Ability and activity vary among people in their 70s, 80s and 90s just as they do earlier in life.

Evidence is piling up that most of our mental skills remain intact as long as our health does, if we keep mentally and physically active. Much of our fate is in our own hands, with "use it or lose it" as the guiding principle. We are likely to slow down in some ways, but there is evidence that healthy older people do a number of things better than young people.

Psychologist James Birren, dean of the Andrus Gerontological Center at the University of Southern California, is one of many researchers to show that older people perform tasks more slowly, from cutting with a knife and dialing a telephone to remembering lists. There are numerous theories about what body changes are responsible but no conclusive answers.

More important, slowing down doesn't make much difference in most of what we do. Slower reflexes are certainly a disadvantage in driving an automobile, but for many activities speed is not important. And when it is, there are often ways to compensate that maintain performance at essentially the same level. "An awful lot of what we can measure slows down," says psychologist Timothy Salthouse of the University of Missouri at Columbia, "but it isn't clear that this actually affects the lives of the people we study in any significant way."

As an example, Salthouse cites an experiment in which he tested the reaction time and typing skills of typists of all ages. He found that while the reactions of the older typists were generally slower than those of younger ones, they typed just as fast. It could be that the older typists were even faster at one time and had slowed down. But the results of a second test lead Salthouse to believe that another factor was at work.

When he limited the number of characters that the typists could look ahead, the older typists slowed greatly, while the younger ones were affected much less. "There may be limits, but I'm convinced that the older typists have learned to look farther ahead in order to type as quickly as the younger typists," Salthouse says.

A similar substitution of experience for speed may explain how older people maintain their skills in many types of problem-solving and other mental activity. Because of this, many researchers have come to realize that measuring one area of performance in the laboratory can give only a rough idea of a person's ability in the real world.

As an example, psychologist Neil Charness of the University of Waterloo in Ontario gave bridge and chess problems to players of all ages and ability levels. When he asked the bridge players to bid and the chess players to choose a move or remember board positions, the older players took longer and could remember fewer of the chess positions. But the bids and the moves they chose were every bit as good as those of younger players. "I'm not sure exactly what the compensatory mechanisms are," Charness says, "but at least until the age of 60, the special processes that the older players use enable them to make up for what they have lost in terms of speed and memory ability."

Many researchers now believe that one reason we associate decline with age is that we have asked the wrong questions. "I suspect that the lower performance of older people on many of the tasks we have been testing stems from the fact that they have found that these things are unimportant, whereas young people might enjoy this kind of test because it is novel," says psychologist K. Warner Schaie of Pennsylvania State University. Relying on their experience and perspective, he says, older people "can selectively ignore a good many things."

Memory is probably the most thoroughly studied area in the relationship between age and mental abilities. Elderly men and women do complain more that they can't remember their friends' names, and they seem to lose things more readily than young people. In his book *Enjoy Old Age,* B. F. Skinner mentions trying to do something that one learned to do as a child—folding a piece of paper to make a hat, for example—and not remembering how. Such a failure can be especially poignant for an older person.

But the fact is that much of memory ability doesn't decline at all. "As we get older, old age gets blamed for problems that may have existed all along," says psychologist Ilene Siegler of the Duke University Medical Center. "A 35-year-old who forgets his hat is forgetful," she says, "but if the same thing happens to grandpa we start wondering if his mind is going." If an older person starts forgetting things, it's not a sure sign of senility or of Alzheimer's disease. The cause might be incorrect medication, simple depression or other physical or mental problems that can be helped with proper therapy.

Psychologists divide memory into three areas, primary, secondary and tertiary. Primary or immediate memory is the kind we use to remember a telephone number between the time we look it up and when we dial it. "There is really little or no noticeable decline in immediate memory," according to David Arenberg, chief of the cognition section at the Gerontology Research Center at the National Institute on Aging. Older people may remember this type of material more slowly, but they remember it as completely as do younger people.

Secondary memory, which, for example, is involved in learning and remembering lists, is usually less reliable as we get older, especially if there is a delay between the learning and the recall. In experiments Arenberg has done, for example, older people have a difficult time remembering a list of items if they are given another task to do in between.

Even with secondary memory, however, where decline with age is common, the precise results depend on exactly how memory is tested. Psychologist Gisela Labouvie-Vief of Wayne State University in Detroit has found that older people excel at recalling the metaphoric meaning of a passage. She asked people in their early 20s and those in their 70s to remember phrases such as "the seasons are the costumes of nature." College students try to remember the text as precisely as they can. Older people seem to remember the meaning through metaphor. As a result, she says, "they are more likely to preserve the actual meaning, even if their reproduced sentence doesn't exactly match the original." In most situations, understanding the real meaning of what you hear or read is more important than remembering the exact words.

Part of the problem with tests of memory is that most match older people against students. "As long as we accept students as the ideal, older people will look bad," Labouvie-Vief says. Students need to memorize every day, whereas most older people haven't had to cram for an exam in years. As an example of this, psychologist Patricia Siple and colleagues at Wayne State University found that older people don't memorize as well as young students do. But when they are matched against young people who are not students, they memorize nearly as well.

The third kind of memory, long-term remembrance of familiar things, normally decreases little or not at all with age. Older people do particularly well if quickness isn't a criterion. Given time and the right circumstances, they may do even better than younger men and women. When psychologist Roy Lachman of the University of Houston and attorney Janet Lachman tested the ability to remember movies, sports information and current events, older people did much better, probably because of their greater store of information. Since they have more tertiary memory to scan, the Lachmans conclude, older people scan that kind of memory more efficiently.

Psychologist John Horn of the University of Denver and other researchers believe that crystallized knowledge such as vocabulary increases throughout life. Horn, who has studied the mental abilities of hundreds of people for more than 20 years, says, "If I were to put together a research team, I'd certainly want some young people who might recall material more quickly, but I'd also want some older crystallized thinkers for balance."

Researchers often echo the "use it or lose it" idea. When psychologist Nancy Denney of the University of Wisconsin-Madison uses the game "20 questions" in experiments, she finds that the needed skills are not lost. "The older people start off by asking inefficient questions," she says, "but we know that the abilities are still there because once they see the efficient strategy being used by others, they learn it very quickly."

Psychologist Liz Zelinski of the University of Southern California makes a similar point when she tests the ability to read and understand brief passages. People in their 70s and 80s show no significant decline in comprehension. "Our tests don't involve the kind of questions that require older people to store information temporarily in memory," she cautions. "Tests like that might show declines." Zelinski has also found that older men and women read her tests just as fast as younger people do. "It is a good guess that they maintain the ability to read quickly because they do it all the time," she says.

Even when skills atrophy through disuse, many people can be trained to regain them. Schaie and psychologist Sherry Willis of Pennsylvania State University . . . reported on a long-term study with 4,000 people, most of whom were older. Using individualized training, the researchers improved spatial orientation and deductive reasoning for two-thirds of those they studied. Nearly 40 percent of those whose abilities had declined returned to a level they had attained 14 years earlier.

Mnemonics is another strategy that can help people memorize something as simple as a shopping list. Arenberg has found that older people are much better at remembering a 16-item list if they first think of 16 locations in their home or apartment and then link each item with a location. With practice, they master this technique very easily, Arenberg says, "and become very effective memorizers."

When it comes to aging's effect on general intelligence, as measured by standard IQ tests, the same questions of appropriateness, accuracy and motivation complicate the findings. Psychologist Paul Costa, chief of the laboratory of personality and cognition of the Gerontology Research Center at the National Institute on Aging in Baltimore, points out that many early studies on aging tested older people and younger people at the same time, instead of testing the same people over a period of years. These studies were, in effect, measuring the abilities of older people, largely lower-income immigrants, against the generations of their children and grandchildren. "The younger people enjoyed a more comfortable life-style, were better educated and didn't face the same kind of life stresses," he says, "so comparisons were mostly inappropriate."

Most researchers today are uncomfortable with the idea of using standard intelligence tests for older people. "How appropriate is it to measure the 'scholastic aptitude' of a 70-year-old?" asks University of Michigan psychologist Marion Perlmutter.

She and others, including Robert Sternberg at Yale, believe that aspects of adult functioning, such as social or professional competence and the ability to deal with one's environment, ought to be measured along with traditional measures of intelligence. "We are really in the beginning stages of developing adequate measures of adult intelligence and in revising what we think of as adult intelligence," Perlmutter says. "If we had more comprehensive tests including these and other factors, I suspect that older people would score at least as well and probably better than younger people."

Erroneous ideas about automatic mental deterioration with age hit particularly hard in the workplace. Although most jobs require skills unaffected by age, many employers simply assume that older workers should be phased out. Psychologists David Waldman and Bruce Alvolio of

Special Cases: The Oldest

One group of particular interest to researchers . . . is those more than 85 years old. There are at least two million Americans in this category, more than 1 percent of the population, and growing faster than any other segment.

Depending upon whom you talk to, this group is called the old old, the oldest old or the extreme aged. More than half live independently, by themselves or with a spouse. And many do more than just live. History and current headlines tell us of extraordinary individuals who have done important work in their ninth decade. Mystery writer Agatha Christie, statesman Konrad Adenauer and cellist Pablo Casals are only three well-known examples.

Other less famous but equally industrious men and women of similar advanced age contribute in their own fields. During the 1950s, gerontologist S. L. Pressey studied the lives of 313 people more than 80 years old whose names he found in newspaper clippings, nursing home records and other random sources. He learned that most were working at least part-time. Two men past the age of 90 were presidents of small-town banks and one nonagenarian woman ran an insurance business. If people are given the opportunity to continue making contributions, Pressey concluded—especially if they work in professional fields or are self-employed—they are likely to do so.

Psychologist Marion Perlmutter has begun to study a group of 80-year-olds to see what keeps them going and what we can learn from them to help others. The first interviews suggest that the abilities to be open to new situations and cope with challenges distinguish people who grow during adulthood from people who stabilize or decline. "One reason to study these people is because they're successes. If you make it to 80, you must be doing something right."

the State University of New York at Binghamton recently reviewed 13 studies of job performance and found little support for deterioration of job performance with increasing age. Job performance, measured objectively, increased as employees, especially professionals, grew older. The researchers also discovered, however, that if supervisors' ratings were used as the standard, performance seemed to decline slightly with age. Expectation became reality.

Despite all the experiments and all the talk about gains and losses with age, we should remember that many older people don't want to be compared, analyzed or retrained, and they don't care about being as fast or as nimble at problem solving as they once were. "Perhaps we need to redefine our understanding of what older people can and cannot do," Perlmutter says. Just as children need to lose some of their spontaneity to become more mature, perhaps "some of what we see as decline in older people may be necessary for their growth." While this does not mean that all age-related declines lead to growth or can be ignored, it does highlight a bias in our youth-oriented culture. Why do we so often think of speed as an asset and completely ignore the importance of patient consideration?

Source: Jeff Meer, *Psychology Today* (June 1986), pp. 60–64.

• *Creativity:* It is difficult to define "creative." Some argue that experience often reins in the impulses required for creative thinking. If this is so, older people, who have more life "experience," may not be less able to be creative but may simply be resisting the temptation to be so. [18]

FIGURE 4.4
A Time for Creativity

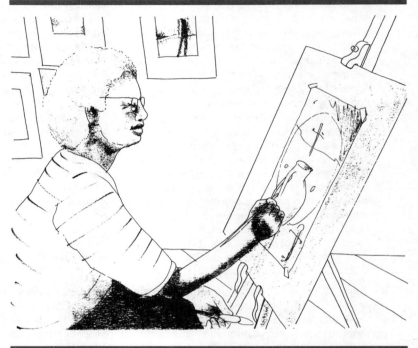

Free of the time constraints and burdens associated with raising a family and earning a living, many older people find new and rewarding outlets for their creativity.

Scientists need to conduct more research in order to reach definitive conclusions about the influence of age on cognitive functioning and on the extent to which these changes stem from physiological and environmental factors. [19] The task is made more difficult by the fact that these changes may result from such external factors as motivation, physical health, and state of mind rather than from the aging process alone. One authority has summarized current findings using the following list:

1. When problem-solving abilities or other intellectual powers diminish before the late 50s, they do so owing to disease and not age.

2. People in their 60s and 70s often suffer a normal decline in some but not all cognitive abilities. This decline affects some but not all individuals. Beyond 80, most people suffer some sort of decline in cognitive ability.

3. People in their 50s may begin to suffer a decrease in their ability to perceive or respond quickly to mental observations.

4. People with severe cardiovascular conditions may find that many of their cognitive abilities decline dramatically during their late 50s or early 60s.

5. Because social and cultural changes are now occurring at such a rapid pace, many people in their late 50s sometimes start feeling as though they have outlived their usefulness to society. This occurs even among those who are currently functioning as well as they ever have, no matter what their age, and is more a matter of perspective. This sense of uselessness is our society's misperception and not a consequence of aging.

6. It is important to distinguish between such faulty thinking, which can often be overcome by reevaluating ourselves, and physiological decline, which may require medical attention and drug therapy. [20]

The most healthy response anyone can have as he or she approaches old age is to choose to keep active—both mentally and physically. Changes in cognitive functioning do occur, and all people will eventually suffer some decline, provided they live long enough. But keeping happy psychologically—just as keeping as physically active and healthy as possible—can delay and often minimize many life changes. **W**

Did You Know That . . .

One recent survey showed that as many as 44 percent of Americans over age 45 fear they will get Alzheimer's disease, when, in actuality, less than 5 percent will have even mild impairment of their faculties.

5

Aging and Mental Health

WHEN SAM RETIRED, his company threw him an elaborate party and gave him a gold watch. The men and women in his office slapped him on the back as they bid him farewell. "Retirement isn't the end of the world," they reminded him. "Drop back in here whenever you feel like it." They assured him that they would always be happy to take a few minutes off to chat with him. Sam thanked them all. Then, with a twinkle in his eye, he said, "One thing, though. Don't sit around waiting for me to 'drop by.' I'm going to be too busy having fun to bother checking up on all of you." [1]

Sam is an elder who is clearly enjoying his later years. In order to have reached old age, he has adapted successfully to numerous, often substantial, changes in his life. Such adaptation is, by definition, one aspect of sound mental health. Contrary to popular belief, maintaining one's mental health in old age is both possible and likely.

Aging can, however, result in certain specific complications that disrupt cognitive functioning. Knowing what these complications are—and how to recognize their symptoms—can make coping with their consequences an easier task for both the sufferer and the caretaker.

Every examination of the effects of aging on mental health requires a discussion of the differences between functional disorders and organic disorders. Both can impair our mental health, but their similarities end there. Our discussion will focus upon 2 conditions that many encounter as they age: depression, a functional disorder, and Alzheimer's disease, a chronic organic disorder.

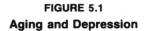

FIGURE 5.1
Aging and Depression

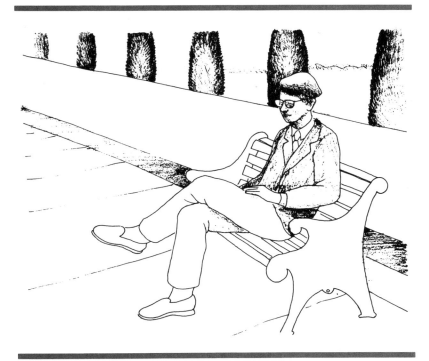

Loneliness and depression can be a major difficulty for some older people. Many factors, such as retirement, widowhood, and chronic or terminal illness, may contribute to feelings of despair and isolation.

FUNCTIONAL DISORDERS

Functional disorders are mental conditions that have no identifiable organic cause; that is, they are not caused by a physical abnormality, disease, or injury. Such disorders include **depression**, anxiety, hypochondria, delusions, compulsions, phobias, and certain types of neuroses. [2] Depression, the most common functional disorder associated with aging, is a morbid state of mind characterized especially by feelings of sadness, dejection, and melancholy that last an abnormally long time or are unreasonable in proportion to the cause.

Functional disorder: A mental or emotional disorder that cannot be associated with a known physical cause.

Depression: A mental state, characterized by extreme sadness or dejection, that persists for an extended period of time.

(continued on p. 90)

Depression: Lifting the Cloud

If you had an ulcer or were disabled by arthritis, you would certainly seek medical help. If back pain kept you in bed, you probably wouldn't hesitate to call your doctor. However, less than 25% of the more than 10 million Americans who suffer from depression ever seek treatment—even though, according to a study by the Rand Corporation, depression is *more* disabling than arthritis, ulcers, diabetes, or high blood pressure. It is as serious as emphysema or back problems in limiting people in their physical activities and confining them to bed. In fact, only heart pain and advanced coronary artery disease more severely limit such activities as dressing, bathing, walking, or playing sports.

Whether it is fear of social stigma, fear that they are going crazy or a belief that "you just need to pull yourself up by your bootstraps," too many people suffer needlessly from depression. True depression is a medical condition, and more than 80% of all cases of it can be successfully treated.

Making the diagnosis
Virtually all healthy people will experience the "blues"—a short-term dip in mood that lifts when a person's outlook improves—at some time in life. Nearly everyone, too, will experience deep and abiding grief at the death of a spouse or child or other tragic life event—grief that may take a long time to pass. Clinical depression (see "The telltale signs"), however, is a medical illness, without an apparent immediate cause, that does not lift when circumstances change, that can last for several months or years, and that can lead to suicide.

There are several different types of mood disorders, of which major, or unipolar, depression is the most common. In the course of a lifetime, 25% of the population will suffer at least one major depressive episode.

Bipolar—or manic-depressive—disorder is a less common form, in which a patient alternates between depressive and expansive emotional states. Manic episodes can include euphoria, hyperactivity, excessive energy, insomnia, hallucinations, and sometimes violent or reckless behavior.

Many people do not recognize the symptoms of depression in themselves—or, if they do, they think they have a character flaw rather than an illness. Then, too, the feelings of hopelessness and lack of vitality that are the very symptoms of depression may keep people from seeking medical help.

In older people especially, "masked" or unrecognized depression (complaints of aches and pains or listlessness that they and others might attribute to aging or to simple hypochondria) is common. But it is never normal to feel unhappy all the time as you get older.

A combination of causes
The cause of depression is elusive—and it is clear that successful treatment must take into account the whole fabric of a person's life, not just a single thread. While there is speculation that a complex interweaving of biology, personality, and inadequate or inappropriate coping strategies that a person has developed over the course of a lifetime leads to depression, there is no evidence that any of these alone can cause mood disorders.

It is thought that a disruption in the normal interplay between certain chemicals in brain cells and the neurotransmitters (substances that facilitate the passage of impulses from one nerve cell to another) plays an important part in the onset of clinical depression. Depression also runs in families (although some experts assert that this is due to a learned coping style rather than a genetic trait). Studies of identical twins, for example, show that if one twin suffers from depression, there is a 50-to-90% chance that the other twin will, too. A 1987 study seemed to find a single gene for manic-depression that ran through six generations of an Amish family—but follow-up analyses have since raised serious doubts as to whether any single gene could account for any kind of depression.

Since not every pair of identical twins suffers from the same mood disorders, psychological factors presumably come into play also. Traumas such as the loss of a parent during childhood, repeated low-level stressors, rejections, and failures may contribute. And certain personality types—people with low self-esteem or who tend to be dependent on others—are more vulnerable to depression.

Finally, some cases are rooted in underlying medical conditions: stroke, thyroid disorders, hepatitis, viral pneumonia, or cancer. Other cases are induced by medication, including barbiturates, tranquilizers, heart drugs, hormones, blood pressure medication, pain killers, arthritis drugs, and even some antibiotics. The depression disappears when the medication is stopped. Depression can also be related to chronic alcohol use.

Treatment options

A recent study published in the *Archives of General Psychiatry* found that serious symptoms of depression were completely eliminated within 16 weeks in 50 to 60% of the 250 patients involved—whether they received interpersonal psychotherapy (concentrating on the formation of personality from earliest childhood), cognitive behavioral therapy (concentrating on altering learned behavior patterns), or an antidepressant drug. Of the three treatments, the drug therapy was the quickest—not to mention the cheapest. However, this advantage may be outweighed in cases of minor depression by the side effects of medications.

There are more than 20 antidepressant drugs currently available. They work by modifying the levels of specific neurotransmitters in the brain. Because a variety of drugs target different neurotransmitters, and because imbalances of these neurotransmitters can vary from patient to patient, some drugs may be more effective than others for any individual. Sometimes a combination of drugs is best.

• Tricyclic antidepressants (named for the three-ring chain in their chemical structure) or TCAs, such as Pamelor, Norpramin, and Pertofrane, are

The telltale signs

If you have felt any four of these symptoms nearly every day for two weeks or more, you may well be suffering from depression:
• Persistent sadness, anxiety, or "emptiness"
• Hopelessness or pessimism
• Feeling guilty, worthless, or helpless
• Loss of interest in ordinary activities
• Reduced sex drive
• Sleeping too long, too little, or fitfully
• Changes in appetite or weight
• Feeling fatigued or "slowed down"
• Restlessness or irritability
• Recurrent thoughts of death or suicide
• Difficulty concentrating, remembering, making decisions
• Frequent headaches, backaches, digestive trouble, or other chronic pain that doesn't respond to treatment

the preferred drugs for initial treatment. They have been in use since 1957—so their degree of safety is well-known.

Because of the number of TCAs available, your physician may well try several different ones to find the one that has the fewest side effects for you. Though some patients begin to feel better in as little as a week, full benefit may take as long as six weeks.

• Monoamine oxidase inhibitors—or MAOIs—such as Nardil and Parnate, are the second line of drugs tried if TCAs prove ineffective. MAOI users must restrict their diet to avoid sudden potentially life-threatening jumps in blood pressure. Forbidden foods include: smoked meat, aged cheese, pickled fish, red wine, and yogurts with active cultures.

• Lithium carbonate (such as Eskalith or Lithobid) is very effective in the treatment of bipolar mood disorder, and sometimes helpful for people who have only depressive episodes, especially if the drug is added to a TCA.

• Among other drugs now in use are Desyrel, Xanax (which may be useful for moderate depression, though it leads to physical dependence in a significant minority of patients and so is ordinarily only used as a bridge medication until traditional antidepressants begin to work), and Prozac.

Electroconvulsive therapy

For a very small number of extremely depressed or suicidal people, in whom other treatments have failed, electroconvulsive therapy (ECT) is once again coming into widespread use. Unlike the "shock" treatments administered up until the 1950s, before drug therapy largely replaced it, ECT today is usually done under anesthesia, making it painless. A far lower voltage is used now, for a much shorter period of time (about two seconds), and it is usually administered to only one hemisphere of the brain (the non-dominant, usually the right, hemisphere) to minimize memory loss. For reasons that remain unknown, results can be immediate and dramatic. Since relapse is common within six months, however, ECT is usually followed up with a combination of psychotherapy and drug treatment.

Other therapies

Some studies have suggested that exercise will help relieve mild depression. Sleep deprivation (staying up for a 24-hour period) is occasionally helpful, though the depression usually returns within several days. Some recent studies have shown that sitting under extremely bright lights that simulate daylight for a few hours a day—especially during the winter doldrums—may lift a type of depression appropriately called SAD (seasonal affective disorder).

Since the effects of these alternative treatments remain uncertain, however, no one suffering from depression should be lulled into using them as a means of avoiding medical treatment.

The bottom line

For the most sophisticated treatment, a person suffering from depression will do best to find a teaching hospital with a clinic that specializes in treating mood disorders with a combination of psychotherapy and drugs.

Source: *The Johns Hopkins Medical Letter, Health After 50,* November 1990, pp. 4–5.

Depression during one's later life can result from specific life events, adverse social conditions, a chronic major illness, or even a general decline in health. It can stem from sad or difficult occurrences, such as the death of a loved one or a dramatic reduction in income. [3] Such life events affect people of all ages similarly. But combined with other significant events—say, the prospect of receiving a lower income in addition to a continued sense of loneliness, dependency, or immobility—they may affect older adults more critically. This is especially true of those in their mid-70s and beyond. [4] In many cases, it is the threat of such events as much as their actual occurrence that brings on depression. But depression can be treated.

You may have noticed that a number of the triggering factors mentioned above are related directly or indirectly to physical well-being. Success in preventing the onset of premature major chronic illness in later life, then, not only is worthwhile in its own right but also can help prevent or limit the depression that so often accompanies such events.

ORGANIC DISORDERS

Psychiatrists define an **organic disorder** as a mental or emotional disorder that results from an identifiable physiological cause. Some common symptoms of an organic illness include confusion, memory loss, incoherent speech, and disorientation. There are 2 types of organic disorders: reversible and irreversible.

(continued on p. 96)

FIGURE 5.2
Alzheimer's Disease and Brain Loss

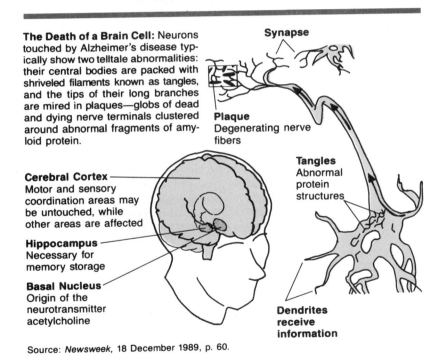

The Death of a Brain Cell: Neurons touched by Alzheimer's disease typically show two telltale abnormalities: their central bodies are packed with shriveled filaments known as tangles, and the tips of their long branches are mired in plaques—globs of dead and dying nerve terminals clustered around abnormal fragments of amyloid protein.

Synapse

Plaque
Degenerating nerve fibers

Cerebral Cortex
Motor and sensory coordination areas may be untouched, while other areas are affected

Tangles
Abnormal protein structures

Hippocampus
Necessary for memory storage

Basal Nucleus
Origin of the neurotransmitter acetylcholine

Dendrites receive information

Source: *Newsweek,* 18 December 1989, p. 60.

The brain contains billions of neurons, which form an intricate electrochemical circuit. Normal brain function requires that various neuron groups produce particular chemical transmitters and that the transmitters pass freely between individual cells. The dementia associated with Alzheimer's is caused by a breakdown of this transmission system. When neurons based in the basal nucleus fail to distribute the acetylcholine into the hippocampus and cerebral cortex, memory and other mental functions suffer.

Organic disorder: A mental or emotional disorder that results from an identifiable physical cause.

Toward a Future With Memory

The 51-year-old woman's first signs of trouble, according to her physician, were feelings of jealousy toward her husband. From this somewhat unremarkable (and possibly justified) condition followed other, more baffling personality changes, including fears that someone wanted to kill her, outbursts of loud shrieks and bouts of forgetfulness.

She carried household objects back and forth, hiding them for no apparent reason. Sometimes she got lost in her own apartment.

The woman's five-year decline into full-blown dementia and death, along with autopsy results, were described by her physician in a 1907 medical journal. Though insightful, his report was hardly revolutionary. The physician, a German psychiatric neurologist named Alois Alzheimer, had little reason to suspect that his name would someday become a household word.

But in a modern world with an unprecedented and still-growing number of elderly people, the syndrome he so carefully documented in a handful of prematurely senile patients has mushroomed into a global health crisis, affecting as many as 4 million individuals in the United States alone. Alzheimer's disease, asserts T. Franklin Williams, director of the National Institute on Aging in Bethesda, Md., "is by far the most threatening epidemic that we have in our nation."

Recent estimates suggest the disorder may affect almost half of the U.S. population aged 85 and older. It costs the nation nearly $90 billion each year and takes an immense emotional toll on its victims and their family members. Eight of the institutes and divisions within the National Institutes of Health now sponsor or conduct research on the debilitating disease.

Yet after more than a decade of intensive research, scientists for the most part remain puzzled as ever. Indeed, to diagnose Alzheimer's, doctors today rely upon essentially the same behavioral and biological hallmarks described by Alzheimer himself more than 80 years ago: a progressive dementia including severe loss of memory; and the accumulation in brain tissue of protein deposits called amyloid plaques, recognizable only upon autopsy.

Scientists have amassed an immense amount of information—"too *many* clues," in the words of one Alzheimer's specialist—about the biochemistry behind these classic symptoms. The accumulating knowledge hints that investigators may eventually solve the Alzheimer's riddle, perhaps by the end of the century, some say.

But daunting hurdles remain, according to Alzheimer researchers who gathered recently at the National Institutes of Health to pool their findings. Scientists at the meeting proposed causes ranging from mitochondrial mutations to unidentified, blood-borne agents, and potential cures ranging from simple aspirin to overlapping doses of potent, synthetically produced brain chemicals.

Faced with a plethora of possibilities, researchers admit they simply don't know what's at the root of the disease. And with no clear idea about the fundamental differences between Alzheimer's disease and normal aging—nor any reliable animal model upon which to try novel treatments—they say they remain hobbled in their attempts to develop effective treatments or preventive measures. Standard treatment today is limited to antidepressants and other drugs that target secondary symptoms of the disease.

"In order to prevent a disease, we generally need to understand its cause. And we certainly don't know the cause of Alzheimer's," says Leon Thal, a neuroscientist at the University of California, San Diego.

Until recently, experimental treatments for Alzheimer's have focused on the most prominent biological deficit associated with the disease: the death of nerve cells that secrete the neurotransmitter acetylcholine in the brain. These so-called cholinergic neurons constitute some of the main lines of communication between the forebrain and the hippocampus, two brain areas responsible for higher cognitive functions and memory.

Early attempts to maintain acetylcholine levels

by providing two of the compound's raw ingredients—choline and lecithin—had essentially no effect in Alzheimer's patients. More recently, researchers have focused on such drugs as physostigmine and tetrahydroaminoacridine (THA), which help prevent acetylcholine breakdown and thus may help patients make the most of the limited acetylcholine supplies they still possess.

So far, about 125 Alzheimer's patients have received physostigmine, with mixed results. New analogs of the drug—which remain active in the body longer than the two hours typical of the original form—may prove somewhat more effective, researchers say.

THA, which stirred controversy in 1987 when the Food and Drug Administration called into question the methodology used by the drug's primary investigator, remains "interesting and promising" despite some evidence that it may cause short-term liver toxicity, says Thal. A three-year, multicenter U.S. trial of the drug [was] scheduled for completion [late in 1990].

But attempts to alleviate Alzheimer's symptoms by manipulating the cholinergic system are hampered by scientists' incomplete understanding of how the complex system operates. Moreover, says Israel Hanin of Loyola University in Chicago, "it's increasingly clear that the cholinergic system itself is not the Lone Ranger of Alzheimer's disease, and that other neurotransmitter systems are involved."

A handful of Alzheimer researchers have begun exploring the potential roles of other neurotransmitter systems, including the noradrenergic and serotonergic networks in the brain. Others, however, suspect that the real heart of the disease lies beyond the brain and that neuronal death represents a secondary or even tertiary "side effect" of a more fundamental dysfunction. Several intriguing theories along these lines are today drawing research attention.

Mitochondrial mischief: Some researchers propose that at least some cases of Alzheimer's may result from an inherited defect in mitochondria, the oxygen-dependent energy factories in cells. Mitochondria contain proteins essential to normal metabolism, and an inherited defect in these proteins could lead to the production of toxic, metabolic by-products or oxidizing "free radicals" that could damage neurons in the brain. Even if the mitochondrial defect were found in all cells, the resulting metabolic inefficiency might affect neurons more than it would other cells, since neurons require extraordinarily large amounts of oxygen.

The evidence for mitochondrial involvement in Alzheimer's is sketchy but provocative. Mitochondria within the protein plaques deposited on and around neurons in Alzheimer brains appear abnormal in photomicrographs, and evidence indicates they process oxygen with less than their usual amount of vigor in these patients.

Even more compelling, genetic analysis of mitochondria in the blood platelets of Alzheimer's patients reveals DNA mutations that appear capable of disrupting normal mitochondrial metabolism. W. Davis Parker Jr. of the University of Colorado Health Sciences Center in Denver says he has found "heavy hits," or mutations, in the mitochondrial DNA of five of the six living Alzheimer's patients he examined. He suggests that Alzheimer's, which in most cases seems to lack a hereditary pattern, might be inherited through mitochondrial DNA, which comes only from the mother. (Most genes are inherited through the DNA in cell nuclei, which comes from both parents.) Scientists have tentatively linked other "late onset" diseases to mitochondrial defects, he notes. And because of their complex inheritance pattern, maternally derived traits can give the appearance of arising sporadically in the population.

If Alzheimer's results from mitochondrial malfeasance, researchers might possibly treat or prevent it with drugs such as co-enzyme Q and deprenyl, which can suppress oxidative damage, Parker suggests. Others note that a synthetic version of a naturally occurring substance called acetyl-L-carnitine appears promising in its ability to both enhance cholinergic function and prevent oxidative damage.

Membrane defects: Noting that "neurons are mostly membranes," Richard J. Wurtman of the Massachusetts Institute of Technology in Cambridge calls the study of membranes "the wave of the future" in Alzheimer's research. Membranes are mostly lipids, he says, and some of the latest thinking suggests the disease might result from abnormalities in certain membrane lipids.

Jay W. Pettegrew, a neuroscientist at the University of Pittsburgh, uses nuclear magnetic resonance spectroscopy to examine debris from cell-membrane breakdown in the brains of living Alzheimer's patients. The noninvasive technique allows him to detect, over time, any evolving changes in the types of lipid metabolites in the brain.

So far, Pettegrew has noted that the Alzheimer's patients have higher brain levels of lipid metabolites called phosphomonoesters (PMEs) than do people suffering from other kinds of dementia. Interestingly, PME levels increase in the brain of developing fetuses just before an event called programmable cell death—a genetically determined, large-scale massacre of extraneous nerve cells. Alzheimer's might represent a replay of this early genetic program, Pettegrew suggests.

Moreover, he says he's "intrigued" that the three-dimensional structures of PMEs closely resemble those of certain neurotransmitters, suggesting PMEs could trigger their own signals in the brain. "They look the same," he says, "but do they act the same?" If PMEs do cause damage by binding to neurotransmitter receptors in the brain, then perhaps specific receptor blockers, such as those currently under investigation in stroke patients, may prove useful against Alzheimer's disease, Pettegrew says.

Protein problems: Dennis Selkoe of Harvard University proposes another way in which membrane abnormalities could play a role in Alzheimer's. He focuses on beta amyloid, the primary protein that accumulates in Alzheimer brains. Beta amyloid, he notes, is actually a snippet of protein cleaved from a much larger protein called amyloid precursor protein (APP), which sticks out from cell membranes. Normally, APP's cleavage site remains well protected, buried within the lipid matrix of a cell membrane. One way for APP to lose a beta amyloid fragment might be for the membrane to leave that key cleavage site ex-

posed to enzyme activity, perhaps because of a structural defect in the membrane.

Moreover, with the [1989] detection of amyloid deposits not just in the brain but in many parts of Alzheimer patients' bodies, Selkoe proposes that the beta amyloid associated with Alzheimer's may originate somewhere else in the body, with the protein deposits later accumulating in the blood vessels, brain and elsewhere. He points to evidence of a similar genesis for other, apparently related diseases called amyloidoses, all of which involve the production of abnormal protein fragments and their deposition in tissues.

Therapeutic approaches worth investigating for such a mechanism include drugs that block the APP-cleaving enzyme or antibody-like substances that could "mop up" the amyloid protein fragments before they begin to accumulate in the brain.

Immune reactions: At some point in Alzheimer's disease, the immune system gets involved. But scientists remain uncertain whether the disease is itself an immune disorder or whether the immune system joins the fray late in the biochemical process.

In studies of Alzheimer brains, researchers have noted that microglial cells—"housekeeping" cells within the brain—often contain bits of neuronal debris. But do they themselves start the trouble by imprudently gobbling up innocent neurons, or are the microglial cells simply cleaning up another troublemaker's mess?

Whatever starts it, once microglial cells consume these neuronal tidbits they can produce a molecule called HLA that attracts white blood cells called T-lymphocytes and stirs them into a hyperactive state. This finding, along with controversial evidence that Alzheimer's patients harbor antibodies against their own brain tissue, leaves many researchers looking at the immune system as a key participant in the pathology.

"Our hypothesis is that there is a specific immune response against yet-to-be-identified antigens in Alzheimer's disease brains," says Felicia Gaskin, a behavioral neurobiologist at the University of Virginia in Charlottesville. It remains unclear whether those antigens are infectious particles such as viruses or are the patient's own proteins triggering an autoimmune response, she and others say. For that matter, any of several immune-cell stimulants may trigger Alzheimer's, says Joseph Rogers of the Institute for Biogerontology Research in Sun City, Ariz. "I think all you need are a few activated lymphocytes wandering into the brain . . . and away you go."

Henry M. Wisniewski of the New York State Institute for Basic Research in Developmental Disabilities, in Staten Island, also blames the immune system for many of the problems in the disease. But he suggests that immune-system scavenger cells in the brain may directly contribute to the Alzheimer's scenario by overproducing beta amyloid themselves.

On the other hand, says William R. Markesbery of the University of Kentucky in Lexington, perhaps researchers should blame the immune system not for overactivity but instead for loafing on the job when it ought to be disposing of the accumulating bits of beta amyloid. "Amyloid deposition may represent a failure of the sanitation department," he says.

Whatever its role in the disease, the immune system clearly becomes activated at some point, triggering an inflammatory process that would best be shut down, says Patrick L. McGeer of the University of British Columbia in Vancouver. Toward that end, he proposes a simple addition to the Alzheimer's armamentarium: aspirin.

McGeer cites his own anecdotal evidence that Alzheimer's rarely strikes rheumatoid arthritis patients, who typically take aspirin on a regular basis. "An aspirin a day keeps the gerontologist away," he suggests. Other researchers have reported observations that contradict McGeer's, and they note that even if aspirin had potential in Alzheimer's, it might not enter the brain in sufficient concentrations before reaching toxic levels in the blood.

Other theories on Alzheimer's genesis abound. Researchers still wonder, for example, whether aluminum—found in high concentrations in amyloid plaques—helps cause the syndrome or simply becomes concentrated in these protein deposits later in the disease.

And scientists have yet to understand the differences between familial Alzheimer's—the clearly inherited form accounting for an apparent minority of cases—and noninherited Alzheimer's, which appears unpredictably in the elderly and somewhat more frequently in women than in men.

Meanwhile, efforts to evaluate new therapies remain hampered by the lack of a clear biological marker allowing physicians to diagnose the disease before the patient's death, by the uncertain value of various cognitive tests used to measure improvements in patients' behavior and memory, and by the difficulty of finding enough study participants with Alzheimer's who are not already taking many other drugs.

And, as with all diseases of the central nervous system, drug developers must wrestle with the problem of getting their product into the brain, past the membranous border patrol known as the blood-brain barrier. All told, says James Simpkins of the University of Florida in Gainesville, "Alzheimer's disease is probably more difficult to treat pharmaceutically than any other disease."

Nonetheless, asserts Williams of the National Institute on Aging, "the scientific base is there" to devise an effective treatment. With more than a dozen drugs already in clinical trials and with drug companies using automated methods capable of screening hundreds of compounds per week for potential nervous-system activity, "we can do it within the next five or 10 years if we want to," he declares.

Even a drug capable of delaying the onset of Alzheimer's by a decade or two would be a worthy goal, says Thal, who adds wryly: "That would allow us to die quietly and nicely from some other disease."

Source: Rick Weiss, *Science News* Vol. 137 (February 24, 1990), pp. 120–123.

Reversible organic disorders may occur as a side effect of medications; as a symptom of an imbalanced metabolic condition such as hypoglycemia, acute emotional stress, vitamin deficiencies, or malnutrition; or may accompany certain diseases of the gastrointestinal, hepatic (liver), cardiac, or vascular systems. [5]

Irreversible chronic disorders, or **senile dementia**, are characterized by gradual and permanent deterioration of mental functions. Such conditions are divided into 2 categories: those caused by the deterioration of brain tissue, such as **Alzheimer's disease**, and those caused by an interruption of the blood supply to the brain, such as **cerebral atherosclerosis**. [6] Scientists estimate that as many as 15 percent of people over 65 have senile dementia to some degree. Alzheimer's disease claims 40 percent of geriatric patients who suffer dementia.

Alzheimer's Disease

The disease we know as Alzheimer's disease was named for the German neurobiologist Alois Alzheimer, who first detected the abnormal microscopic fibers in the brain that characterize the disease. Although scientists have improved their knowledge of Alzheimer's disease dramatically since the mid-1970s, they still do not know what exactly causes it or how to cure this degenerative illness. They have, however, been able to pinpoint the stages of the disease, which are as follows:

1. Forgetfulness, a loss of recent memory, a lessening of emotional responses, and disorientation.

2. An increase in forgetfulness accompanied by a deterioration of higher learning functions.

3. Complete disorientation resulting in helplessness and total dependency.

Treatment for Alzheimer's disease at present is limited to medications that quell some of the symptoms that are indirectly related to the disease, such as depression and anxiety. These therapies cannot stop the disease from its ultimately destructive path, but they do lessen its impact on both the sufferers and those who care for them. [7]

LIMITING THE MENTAL EFFECTS OF AGING

Some researchers insist that psychological and social adjustments are more important to a long life than biological factors.

"You can eat and drink all the right things," they argue, "refrain from eating and drinking all the wrong things, take all the right supplements, and still not thrive *if*, for instance, you smoke, never fasten the seat belt in your car, lead a totally sedentary life, are depressed and pessimistic, have no friends or social support network, are bored, [or] have nothing and no one you care very much about." [8]

Because it is often so difficult to measure the many aspects of mental functioning and because each aspect is so interrelated, pinpointing the mental consequences of aging is an inexact science at best. As you might expect, then, developing some formula or recipe for maintaining your mental health throughout life and into old age is also difficult. But people who seek

(continued on p. 102)

Productive Aging and the Future of Retirement

What will be the productive economic potential of older persons in the future aging society? Can the aging hope to make meaningful and significant contributions to both economic and social productivity as we approach and enter the twenty-first century? What are the forces that will affect this potential and what are the key choices that society must make to achieve a productive aging society?

These concerns, along with growing interest in employment alternatives by some older persons, are leading some to challenge the traditional meaning of "retirement" as a complete cessation from work and to suggest that retirement may become an inappropriate description of future societal patterns; that is, in the future the meaning of retirement will change or a different social definition of aging will be needed.

After many years of effort and many social policy decisions, we have clearly developed an extremely beneficial set of choices for older persons which allow most to limit or entirely refrain from work if they choose to do so. As it turns out, some of our policies may have caused the pendulum to swing too far away from productivity in favor of leisure life-styles for the aging. However,

a reversal of the pendulum in the opposite direction is not necessarily desirable either, and clearly would not be a popular policy for most older people today.

Thus, in considering the future productive roles of older people, it is important to clarify views of work and retirement based on both today's actual circumstances, which of course are influenced by past policies, and tomorrow's possible trends which can be influenced by future policies.

A frequent misconception is to consider the decisions that older people make regarding retirement as "point-in-time" choices that are made based on immediate circumstances near the time of retirement. In reality, retirement decisions are influenced by *life-cycle circumstances* of people, including concerns about health, economic status, personal priorities, and public and private sector policies that have, over time, conditioned their understanding of the choices actually available for them. If these factors change, then the timing and content of retirement and employment decisions may change as well. In general, the overall economy and the incentives of public and private pension plans will continue to significantly influence the choices of older people both today and in the future.

Thus, to understand what may occur in the years ahead that might encourage economic productivity by older persons, it is necessary to consider how the current pattern of retirement developed, the factors that influence and determine today's early retirement patterns, and whether any flexibility in retirement could be introduced in the future that would encourage and enable more older persons to be productive?

The Changing Meanings of 'Retirement'

In today's society, "retirement" clearly has multiple meanings and it is no longer a safe assumption that someone who either says he is retired or is classified as retired, does not work. Yet, since less than 3 percent of the entire work force of the United States are aged 65 and above and those 55–64 represent only 11 percent of American workers, there is a clear connection between retirement and a nonemployed status.

At the initiation of the Social Security Program in 1935, age 65 was considered "normal" retirement age, and as retirement became more and more institutionalized over time, most workers came to accept and expect retirement as an important portion of their lifetime. It was clearly recognized at the beginning of the Social Security program that the goal of American retirement policy was to provide a period of leisure (or rest) after the conclusion of working life. While it took some time to make this goal a realistic possibility for many Americans, its achievement, notably in the last 25 years, certainly is considered a major accomplishment of United States' policy for the aging.

Therefore, the major pattern since the passage of Social Security in 1935 has been decreasing employment of the aging and, in fact, an acceleration of this trend in the last 20 years, particularly because of the earlier availability of pension income. Both federal and private sector policies influence the timing of retirement decisions, and today, the key provisions of these policies allow workers to receive pension benefits at early ages—and when benefits are offered, most older persons accept them readily. On the other hand,

few government or private sector policies provide incentives for older persons to either remain at work after pension benefits become available or return to work after receiving benefits.

There are some recent developments that could slightly alter the current relatively rigid retirement programs. Probably the most important of these changes is the fact that nearly 25 percent of all people who begin receiving Social Security benefits now continue to work for short periods of time—usually one to three years. This indicates that acceptance of pension benefits need not mean complete withdrawal from the labor force. In addition, it now appears that the decline in the number of younger people entering the work force between now and the early part of the next century (the "baby-bust" generation) will produce some shortages of workers and that it may be possible to draw older workers back into the work force to meet such labor demands.

Older worker employment service programs, notably *Operation ABLE* (Ability Based on Long Experience) and *SCORE* (Service Corps of Retired Executives), now located in many major metropolitan areas of the United States, have been increasingly successful in placing older workers into jobs. (A federally supported project, the Senior Community Service Employment Program, also has successfully assisted significant numbers of lower-income older persons to secure productive employment.) In fact, in many areas where these programs operate, the demand for workers now exceeds the supply of older persons willing to be employed. (However, most of the jobs being offered are relatively low-paying service positions.)

Recently, these private older-worker employment programs have reported that many more older job seekers with substantial education and experience are seeking postretirement jobs, but that employers either do not have these jobs or do not offer vacant high level positions to these job seekers. This is one aspect of a general problem in the United States—too-limited development of flexible work schedules for older workers. With a few notable exceptions, employers have not modified their employment policies in ways that would be attractive to older workers who usually are interested in part-time employment on flexible schedules and where earnings remain below the Social Security earnings test level. A small number of employers have experimented very successfully with specialized policies for older workers and have been able to rehire or newly hire significant numbers of experienced and productive employees. Despite significant efforts to publicize these programs, they have not been widely replicated. This is understandable since many organizations have been reducing their staffs through offering early retirement and most recognize that today's pension policies are not designed to encourage employment after retirement. Unless a particularly serious labor shortage exists or develops, it is not very likely that business organizations will choose to focus on policies to attract older workers. This does not mean that firms are opposed to older employees per se, but rather that they do not believe that these workers represent a significant labor supply pool or that older workers can be easily motivated to return to employment.

Under these circumstances, does "retirement" have only one meaning—complete cessation of economic productivity? Until recently, the unequivocal answer to this question was yes. But now, with more people continuing employment after receiving pension benefits and the number of specialized older-worker employment programs growing, the definition of retirement is beginning to change toward "pension recipient"—which does not automatically imply that a person in this status has no connection with the work force. This more neutral term is a more realistic definition of today's circumstances, where pensions are available after varying lengths of employment and are sometimes provided to persons as early as age 40. What we are beginning to observe therefore are changes in the way aging itself is both defined and viewed by society.

Pensions have historically been related to age because typically, to receive a pension, a person must work for many years and thus becomes "older." And it has been assumed (and is still accepted) that pension receipt and retirement—

meaning complete cessation of work—are synonymous. But in aging societies such as those of Western Europe, Japan, and the United States, where life expectancy continues to increase, the meaning of retirement can change or its definition can become more flexible so that being retired (or receiving a pension) no longer means that a person is not economically productive or, more important, is not *expected* to be productive. The fact that despite enjoying their retirement, between one-third and one-half of today's retirees report that they would prefer to work (usually part-time) clearly indicates that in their view, retirement is not necessarily a period where work should not be performed. If more opportunities were actually available, no doubt more older people would work.

The key issues are:
• Will today's early retirement policies continue, and if they do, will future older workers leave the labor force entirely and permanently once pensions are available?
• Will different retirement policies be adopted in the future that will provide effective incentives for persons to work at older ages; that is, will flexible policies be implemented to increase labor force participation by older workers?

In the near term then, long before the major growth of the aging population begins in 2010, the youth population will be declining, the middle-aged population increasing, and the older population growing slowly. From a demographic perspective, these circumstances could be conducive for encouraging more economic productivity by older workers over the next 20 years, assuming that employment growth and demand are maintained. But to achieve this goal of productive aging, both public and private policies will have to be modified to encourage older people to either continue to work longer before accepting pensions or, more likely, to return to work after retiring.

Achieving Productivity—
Whose Responsibility?
If retirement and employment patterns are to change in the years ahead, this will only occur if

government pension policies, employer pension and personnel policies, and the attitudes of older persons also change to provide and support more choices for older persons to remain productive. The trends of an aging but increasingly educated work force and growing costs for supporting a larger retired population will characterize the future in both the short and long term. Yet even when these forces are combined with increasing length of life and continued job opportunities in the economy, we cannot realistically predict growth of economic productivity for the aging population. The key reason these trends will not bring about more productivity is that even taken together, they will not produce major changes in retirement behavior unless public and private policies, as well as the expectations and behavior of older persons themselves, are modified.

What then are the appropriate roles and responsibilities for the government, private employers, and older persons themselves relating to changing future retirement patterns?

First, it is clear that public retirement policy, especially as defined through the Social Security program, will have to change if work at older ages is to be encouraged. Such changes need not fundamentally alter income benefit levels provided to retirees or endanger benefits for persons facing disabling health conditions. Changes such as removing the earnings test penalty, providing more significant "bonus" benefit adjustments for deferred retirement, and delaying full retirement benefits until somewhat later ages, all deserve consideration as possible policy choices to encourage longer labor force participation and/or return to employment by older workers.

Second, employer policies also will have to change in order to assure more employment for older workers in the future. In fact, these changes may be more important than modification in public pension policies in order to encourage later life work for persons eligible to receive private pension benefits. This is the case since the current policy of early provision of private pensions (sometimes with supplements until the time of eligibility for Social Security benefits) strongly encourages early acceptance of pensions and leaving the regular work force long before Social Security eligibility begins.

It is unlikely in the near term that employer pension plans will be changed to provide benefits at *later* ages; however, other approaches, including bonuses for deferral of pension receipt and increases in pensions based on return to work, are certainly feasible—assuming that employers want to retain or rehire older workers. In addition, employers desiring to retain or hire these workers will need to adopt several personnel policy changes including flexible scheduling and part-time work choices, elimination of requirements limiting hours that can be worked in a year (this may also require changes in federal law governing private pension plans), continuation of basic employee benefits for older employees, and possible readjustment of pensions, to account for earnings of older workers.

These changes may not in fact be very hard to implement, as has been demonstrated in part by such companies as Travelers Insurance, Grumman Aerospace, and Lockheed Corporation. Some of these types of changes in fact can benefit other groups of employees, such as women with young children, students, younger entry-level workers, and part-time professionals. Therefore, employers may be able to change personnel policies in ways that will influence multiple groups of employees *including older workers* rather than developing specific older-worker policies and programs. In any event, in order to create conditions more suitable for the aging, employers will need to change both benefit and personnel policies.

And third, assuming public *and* private sector policy changes, there must also be changes in behavior of those older persons receiving Social Security retirement benefits and private pension payments. This means that older people must also shift their view of "retirement" or develop a new concept of "pension recipient" that does not imply complete cessation of productive work. Even though job opportunities may exist with appropriate incentives for older workers and older persons may have the training and experience for such jobs, unless they are interested in working, their employment patterns will not change significantly.

Because our society will experience unprecedented growth in the number of older persons over the next 40 years, it is certainly plausible to assume that the aging of the population represents a special historical situation. And thus far, with a population that is gradually aging, we have developed policies that permit the virtual elimination of employment at older ages while being unable to assure economic sufficiency for older persons. This does not mean of course that other forms of productivity are not available to older people, including volunteer work, care-giving, family support, education, and so forth. However, the emphasis of our current policies is to encourage people to leave employment and not to provide incentives to assist them to return to work.

With increased population aging, the costs of support for the "retired" will become very large and will be magnified further by decreasing mortality rates influenced by better health practices earlier in life and by improved medical technology. While much higher levels of care may be needed for people at the oldest ages, many of those who are younger—for example persons under age 75—will be able to continue active lifestyles and will not be precluded in any major way from productive activity, including working.

Aging and Work in the Twenty-First Century

Even with today's emphasis on early retirement, we do know that older people still have opportunities to be productive. Some are engaged in part- or full-time work; many assist with providing care and support for spouses or other relatives and friends; others volunteer their time in health services, education, and social services. At the same time, millions of Americans of all ages pursue leisure activities of all kinds with pleasure and satisfaction. The retired of course have more time (but not always the resources) to pursue leisure activities. This does not necessarily mean that retirees prefer to spend most of their time in these activities—most report that

this is not their preference. But at present there is so little opportunity or incentive for productive employment that leisure activities are often chosen by older people by default.

The overall evidence indicates that baby boomers who will continue to work will be those who will be in good health, have major interest in working or a high need for additional income, and have skills suited to available jobs. If current retirement policies persist through the time when baby boomers will be receiving pension benefits, then it is unlikely that substantial increases in employment of older ages will occur. But, if a combination of changes in government and employer policies could be gradually introduced, it is possible that baby boomers might increase their labor force participation. The changes that would be most significant in bringing about a new employment and retirement continuum include providing full retirement benefits at later ages; providing pension bonuses for delayed retirement; and creating more flexible employment arrangements coordinated with employee benefit arrangements that protect pension and health benefits, while also encouraging employment. These incentives might be effective for baby boomers, who will clearly be interested in greater flexibility during an extended period of older age. There remains a major question about whether retirement policies will change in these directions. And it is unlikely that anything more than informed speculation is possible about the policies and behavior of people who will retire 30–40 years in the future.

It is probably more important to focus on gradual policy changes that could be introduced between now and the early years of the next century which could create more incentives for older persons to remain at work or return to work after receiving pension benefits. If we are to begin to assure a productive older age, these changes are a social imperative.

Source: Malcolm H. Morrison, *The World & I* (December 1988), pp. 525–531.

treatment for mental-health problems and follow certain basic health principles often enjoy good mental health throughout their life span.

Barriers to Treatment

Unfortunately, people sometimes erect a mental barrier that prevents them from coping effectively with stressful situations or confronting and resolving problems as they arise, either of which, if left unaddressed, can lead to mental-health problems. Some people, for example, have a hard time recognizing and coping with certain changes, such as the following:

- retirement
- relocation
- change in residence
- death of a spouse
- death of a friend
- lowered income
- changing roles and social status

Other events occur in mid-life or later (the 50s, 60s, and 70s) that require further adjustment and adaptation. These include a decreasing level of energy, a loss of sensory function, and confronting one's mortality. So it is vital to adopt a resilient attitude and a flexible life-style that can provide you support regardless of life's course.

Those who do not make these adjustments find that the myths and stereotypes of aging become self-fulfilled prophecies. Often patients—and occasionally, even their health-care professionals—appear willing to accept such situations as memory loss, a decline in intelligence, or reduced sexual activity as inevitable, untreatable aspects of aging. That these assumptions are absolutely *untrue* does not deter victims and professionals alike from reacting to such phenomena with resolute inaction.

"Being old," it has been suggested, "is increasingly a state of mind rather than a biological marker.... frailty, forgetfulness, poor health, isolation, occur to fewer people in their 60s and 70s, and have shifted instead to the very old, those over 85." [9] You will see in chapter 6 that once *you* reach those years, the term "very old" is likely to describe those over 100.

Dealing Effectively With Mental Changes

"Keep up your spirits and that will keep up your bodies," Ben Franklin observed. Today we know that the venerable Mr. Frank-

Are You Preparing for Old Age?

Please complete the following statements. Do your responses seem appropriate to you? Why or why not? How do you think other people your age would respond? How would an elderly person respond?

1. The most important things in life to me right now are _____

2. When I am 70 years old, the most important things to me will probably be _____

3. The things that I look forward to about aging are _____

4. The things that I dread the most about aging are _____

5. If my parents are no longer able to care for themselves, I will _____

6. If I am no longer able to care for myself, I will _____

7. The terms that come to mind when I think of "old" people are _____

8. To ensure that I will live a full and healthy life, I am doing the following things right now _____

Source: Rebecca J. Donatelle et al., *Access to Health* (Englewood Cliffs, NJ: Prentice Hall, 1988), p. 434.

lin understated the case. We acknowledge, in fact, that if you don't keep up your spirits, all the body potions and health remedies you undertake will alone not do the job of keeping up your body. [10]

It may seem obvious as well by now, but perhaps the most important thing a person can do to forestall or combat the mental-health effects of aging is to maintain his or her physical health. One study conducted by the National Institute of Mental Health, for example, compared 2 groups of disease-free men and women between the ages of 60 and 92. One group was designated "extremely healthy"; the other was labeled "merely healthy." Among the findings: Those in the "extremely healthy" group exhibited a cerebral blood flow and oxygen consumption that were equivalent to those of normal persons 50 years younger. The "merely healthy" group tested significantly lower. In addition, the "extremely healthy" group showed only a minimal decline in mental abilities and perceptual functions when compared to the younger controls. [11] Clearly, maintaining health and vigor into old age helps people maintain their mental capacities.

Among the steps you can take to preserve your mental health are these:

- Take an inventory of your strengths and weaknesses. Then, using the approaches outlined in chapter 6, make every effort to enhance your existing strengths, acquire new ones, eliminate or lessen the weaknesses you can modify, and learn to accept the weaknesses you cannot change.
- Develop and maintain a network of family and friends with whom you keep in touch. This skill is especially important later in life when such problems as poor health, limited transportation, and/or financial strain may interfere with your ability to maintain a wide network of contacts. Those who live with others—whether family, friends, or new acquaintances acquired for that purpose—maintain a better state of mental health than those who live alone.
- Learn to enjoy being alone. To do this, you need to have established a personal identity independent of your various social, career, and familial roles. These roles undergo change in later years. Without a sense of self-worth, dealing with changing roles becomes difficult. Recognize that being alone does not mean being lonely; it can be a revitalizing experience, a time for reflection and for clearing your mind of unimportant matters. When you can be comfortable with yourself when you are by yourself, you strengthen your sense of individuality and self-esteem, which makes those inevitable life changes easier. Remember—we are so much more than our various roles.
- Don't stagnate mentally. Learn 'to leisure' with ease, without a sense of guilt. Without work that you feel provides a sense that you are "productive," it is easy to fall victim to loneliness, boredom, and depression. Those who age best tend to be involved with others, to have a variety of interests, and to be curious, flexible, and adaptable. Seek new sources of nurturance and stimulation for your mind.
- Establish a weekly exercise and relaxation routine. Studies show that exercising regularly not only improves physiological and psychological functioning but may enhance cognitive functions and psychomotor performance as well. [12] The benefits of learning how to relax your muscle tensions away are obvious.
- Learn to adjust to whatever life brings you. People who are

(continued on p. 108)

Meet the People Who Never Quit Learning

The average man who retires at age 65 today is apt to live to be 80, and the average woman to be 84. As Dr. John Merritt, chief of geriatric medicine at the Hospital of Saint Raphael [New Haven, CT] says, "That's a lot of life to do a lot of things with. If it's approached positively, it can be a great experience." Lifelong learning is one of the ways older people can keep growing.

Learning isn't just "the three R's." And it's not just teachers, textbooks, and tests. Learning can take place on a nature trail, at an overseas resort, in a classroom, or in a favorite armchair.

But wherever it happens—and whatever its subject—learning is strong medicine.

According to Dr. Harvey Rubin, a member of Saint Raphael's attending staff in psychiatry, lifelong learning can lead to long life.

"The more you do, the better you'll feel and the longer you'll live," he says.

Dr. Rubin points out that continuing learning can "counteract depression, the number-one problem among the elderly. It also counteracts anxiety, boredom, and a preoccupation with physical complaints."

David A. Goldberg, 82, says, "When I'm driving home from my classes at Southern Connecticut State University (SCSU), I see men and women, 65 and older, sitting on the bench, depressed, without a mission, without hope, without a goal. And it's sad. There's so much available to take advantage of, and they miss that."

Mr. Goldberg has firsthand knowledge of the value of lifelong learning: [He was scheduled to] receive his B.A. degree in Political Science from SCSU [in May 1990].

"Education promotes social interaction," explains Dr. David Peterson, professor of gerontology at the University of Southern California. "Usually you get educated in groups, and, for older people, getting out and seeing other people seems to be about as important as the particular content of the course. Just by participating in an activity, you're likely to be more social, happier, and better integrated."

Keeping in touch. Opportunities for social contact are especially important for older persons, who may feel cut adrift due to age-related changes. "Some societal structures drop away after age 65," explains Dr. Carol Dye, a gerontologist at the Veterans' Administration Medical Center in St. Louis, Missouri. She adds that, as older family members and friends die, additional social support networks are lost. Declining physical powers or ill health may also necessitate a change in activities. "Continuing education programs can lessen the negative impacts of these changes," Dr. Dye says.

Diane Gibralter, 74, is a case in point. Before beginning art classes at SCSU seven years ago, Mrs. Gibralter was sure she could never be an artist. But now she has two paintings displayed in her grandson's dorm at Yale University, with a commission to complete a third.

Her art work has become so important to her that when she underwent open-heart surgery and was told the operation had not gone as well as expected, she "sat down and started painting, and I got so involved, I didn't even think about it."

Physical health can even get a boost from learning that involves activities such as folk dancing, tennis, walking, or anything else that, as one retiree puts it, "gets the old body moving."

Lifelong learning can be found in many places, though it's not always officially labeled as such. Churches and synagogues, public school systems, community organizations such as the Red Cross and the YMCA—all sponsor classes for adults.

Many colleges and universities have developed special programs for adults beyond typical college age. In Connecticut, for example, the state university system offers tuition-free classes for those 62 and older. Another notable college-based program for older people is the Elderhostel program.

There's a continuing-education topic to suit just about everyone's taste. A small sampling includes:

- Self-protection
- Money management
- Exercise
- Preventive health care
- Modern languages
- Yoga
- Macrame
- Cooking
- American history
- Needlepoint
- Mathematics
- Art appreciation
- Speed-reading
- Folk music
- Chess
- Car care and repair.

Today, adult learners are one of the fastest-growing segments of the population.

One reason is that people are living longer. Another is the growing number of people in the United States who have completed high school or college.

By 1990, an estimated 50 percent of the population over 65 will be high school graduates. And that, says Dr. Peterson, is one of the most important factors influencing a person's participation in continuing education.

But that doesn't mean only high school or college graduates are eager to learn. Many older people who had to forgo an education due to the Depression or World War II are making up for lost time. So are women who interrupted or postponed their education because of childrearing responsibilities.

Aliss Cunningham, for example, was unable to attend college in her youth because of family finances, but enrolled at SCSU under its tuition-free program for senior citizens . . . [to] receive her B.A. degree in English . . .—at the age of 82. "Should I survive after I graduate, and if I'm on my feet, I'll probably audit some more classes," she says.

Unfortunately, getting older doesn't automatically lead to knowing the facts about aging. Many older people believe that loss of their learning ability is inevitable. They interpret the physical signs of aging, such as fatigue or failing vision, as indications that their intelligence is deteriorating as well. Popular culture—with its stereotypes and jokes about the elderly—reinforces these beliefs.

When surveyed, old and young people alike are apt to agree with the myth that "You can't teach an old dog new tricks." The idea that older people lose their ability to learn is one of the most pervasive—and harmful—myths about older people.

Even worse, the myth is self-perpetuating: Younger people assume that older people can't learn, and relegate them to insignificant roles on the sidelines, where there are few opportunities to learn.

According to Saint Raphael's Dr. Merritt, there is no basis for the myth that older people can't learn. "Except for people who have strictly neurological problems, an older person can assimilate as much overall as a younger person can in the same situation," he says.

In a Duke University Medical Center study of people aged 60 to 94, there was no demonstrable decline in overall ability to learn. The primary change in learning capacity noted in older people is that they take longer to learn something new, compared with their own ability when they were younger or with that of younger people.

According to Dr. Dye, "the hallmark of aging is the slowing of function. The brain is less responsive and less retentive as you grow older. Some of the best memories we have are old memories, because they were put into the brain at a time when it was operating better. As you get older, the things that you put into the brain aren't kept there as well and they're more difficult to get to.

"But that doesn't mean older people can't learn," Dr. Dye hastens to add.

Older people *can* learn, and specific conditions can make learning easier for them.

For one thing, learning is a matter of "using it or losing it," Dr. Dye says. "If you have a lifestyle in which learning and reading and keeping up with current events is the norm, then your ability to learn will be much better than that of a person whose lifestyle is more mentally passive."

Dr. Dye suggests the following practical strategies for older learners:

- Take your time learning the information.
- Take your time "retrieving" or remembering information.
- Break learning into small parts. Learn a little, practice what you've learned, then learn a little more.
- Create a stress-free setting for learning.
- Allow yourself time to sit and think about what you've just learned, without interruptions or distractions.
- Participate actively in learning. Allow time to practice what you've learned. Repeat what you've just heard, and repeat the steps you've just been shown.
- Use rhymes or slogans to help jog the memory.
- Organize what you've learned in ways meaningful to you—through outlines, for example.
- Take notes on what you've heard or read and leave yourself notes about things to do or where to go.

Natalie Felske can attest to the value of these suggestions. Mrs. Felske's hopes for a college education were stymied first by the Depression, then by the beginning of World War II, and then again by her husband's illness. A determined lifelong learner, she is now working toward a degree in English at SCSU.

But first she has to complete a language requirement. Her slight hearing impairment has made it difficult to understand her language instructor and, at age 68, she finds that her retention of new information isn't as sharp as it once was, which makes it difficult to learn new vocabulary words in a foreign language. To conquer these problems, she has devised a system of flash cards for vocabulary words. . . .

These learning aids are important not just for older people themselves, but for people who interact with older people in a professional capacity.

For example, physicians who take their fast-paced, stressful work for granted may be frustrated when older patients can't remember information about medications when it's been given to them hurriedly in a busy clinic and without time to ask questions. But the same individual might have little or no trouble remembering instructions if he received them in a quiet room, was given written notes, allowed to repeat back the information, and encouraged to practice carrying out the instructions with supervision.

Because of the differences in their learning styles, many older learners prefer what is known as "age-segregated" learning, where participants are about the same age, and the specific needs of adult learners can be addressed. Others deliberately seek the challenge of an age-integrated setting.

One such learner is Martha Caesar, who in 1978 became one of the first to take advantage of the free tuition program at SCSU. Mrs. Caesar finds that "one of the really exciting aspects of taking courses is the young people." At 81, Mrs. Caesar boasts, "some of my best friends are 18."

Like many older learners, Mrs. Caesar has found learning is more fun the second time around. She finds that "today, the classroom is freer. There's more give and take. I remember my professors as very austere, maybe because I was young and revered them. Now they are much more approachable."

Lack of pressure is another bonus from learning in later life, since courses can be audited without exams or grades. Mrs. Caesar had vowed, "never, as long as I lived, would I write another paper." She now takes classes that strike her fancy, starting off with geography classes and now exploring Asian religions.

Some older learners find that learning is in some ways easier later in life. David Goldberg notes, for example, that older people may be able to pay more attention in class because they aren't looking at classmates and thinking, "Am I going to be dating her?" or worrying about the college football team. Finding a job after graduation also needn't be a concern, although Mr. Goldberg teases his younger classmates that "when I graduate, you better watch out!" since he might look for a job as a political scientist.

Of course, it's not just the older learners who benefit from "age-integrated" learning. Young students benefit from their older colleagues' years of experience.

Frank Trangese, who has taken classes at SCSU since 1980, finds that, at 73, he can offer a unique perspective in history courses, since he has actually lived many of the events being discussed.

Having resolved that "when I retire, I'm not going to let my brain go blank," Mr. Trangese now takes classes at SCSU, is a coordinator for the campus Elderhostel program, and helps register others in the free-tuition program.

In a similar way, Natalie Felske thinks her age allowed her to serve as a "catalyst for discussion" in her creative writing class. Being older, she could "let her hair down" and share personal stories about her life and family, something the younger students were reluctant to do until she served as a role model.

By sharing ideas, strengths, and experiences, lifelong learners end up teaching as well as learning. And that's an important lesson in itself.

—*Melanie Scheller*

Source: *St. Raphael's Better Health,* November/December 1988, pp. 27–32.

young often strive constantly to improve their self-worth. But those same people find that as they age, a more appropriate attitude may be to seek self-enjoyment rather than self-aggrandizement. Power, wealth, position, and reputation are seldom within our total control, but the ability to enjoy ourselves is. A sense of humor, of joy, will always help us mentally through life's rough spots.

• Accept and adapt positively to the reality of your own eventual death. This is a major task for you as you age. Just as you become more comfortable and relaxed after having been in a foreign country or any unfamiliar place for a while, you can become comfortable with thinking about your own death—by facing your fears, you familiarize yourself with that reality. "The removal of fear, any fear, but especially the fear of death, can powerfully enhance your health and enjoyment of life." [13]

Beyond these steps, a successful, positive, and preventive approach to mental health late in life would embrace these general principles:

1. Diagnosing and treating both physical and mental disorders throughout life as they occur.

2. Seeking needed professional help, including education, counseling, and access to medical and psychiatric care early in life.

3. Identifying the available medical and psychiatric facilities that are attractive, accessible, and truly usable.

FIGURE 5.3
A Time for New Experiences

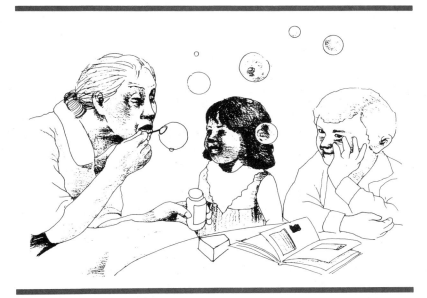

Retirement can be a time of new discoveries and enjoyment. Many people find satisfaction volunteering in their community, such as in a foster grandparent program.

Did You Know That . . .

Modern science is now confirming what French actor and dramatist Jean-Baptiste Molière seemed to know back in the 1600s, when he said in *Love's the Best Doctor,* "The mind has great influence over the body, and maladies often have their origins there."

4. Arranging for the continuity of care appropriate to the rapidly changing needs of an older person.

5. Coordinating the use of professionals from various disciplines who can intervene at all phases of one's life span—who are aware of the issues of aging and the needs of older people and who are able to work effectively with realistic therapeutic and preventive goals, such as modifying one's attitude in the face of mental decline and acceptance of the inevitability of loss and stress in later life. [14]

Add to this the long-standing observation articulated by the psychologist Albert Rosenfeld that "older human beings who maintain a diversity of interests and enthusiasms, and who keep up their supportive social networks, tend to stay healthier and live longer than those who choose to sit around listlessly waiting for the end." [15] Good health adds vigor to all activities, which in turn leads to better mental health, and a fuller life. Ⓦ

6

Influencing the Aging Process

AGING IS A complex process accompanied by many physical and mental changes that occur over a long period of time. Authorities agree that no one theory or "secret" adequately explains the onset, course, and duration of this process. For this reason, there is little anyone can do to extend the absolute human life span. We can, however, extend the number of healthy, vigorous years within that life span. Nearly 70 percent of all deaths are premature. Provided we practice what we already know about health maintenance, many of us can avoid being part of that grim statistic. Our goals of healthful aging, then, are to delay the onset and to minimize the consequences of the aging process.

Ideally, the changes associated with the aging process occur gradually over an extended period of time. If that is so, it becomes much easier to make the physical or behavioral adjustments necessary to minimize the impact of these changes. [1]

Healthful aging does not just happen. It requires planning for our future, something all of us have the capacity to do. According to Paul Insel and Walton Roth, "What you are aiming for now will influence who you are in your 50s, 60s, 70s, and 80s. Flabby muscles, loss of teeth, wrinkles, poor eyesight, stiff joints, failing memory, mental attitude, some chronic diseases—you can control. You can prevent, delay, lessen, even reverse the effects of some deterioration through good health habits [which are] profoundly related to health in later life." [2] Is it too late to begin? Absolutely not. Improving your health habits—specifically those concerning diet, smoking, and alcohol—can make a profound difference at any age. Needless to say, however, the earlier you begin, the better off you are. [3]

Table 6.1 Modifiable Aspects of Aging

Aging Marker	Personal Decision(s) Required
Cardiac reserve	Exercise, nonsmoking
Dental decay	Brushing and flossing, diet
Glucose tolerance	Weight control, diet, exercise
Intelligence tests	Training, practice
Memory	Training, practice
Osteoporosis	Weight-bearing exercise, diet
Physical endurance	Exercise, weight control
Physical strength	Exercise
Pulmonary reserve	Exercise, nonsmoking
Reaction time	Training, practice
Serum cholesterol	Diet, weight control, exercise
Social ability	Practice
Skin aging	Sun avoidance
Systolic blood pressure	Salt limitation, weight control, exercise

Source: J. E. Fries and L. M. Crapo, *Vitality and Aging* (New York: W. H. Freeman and Co., 1981).

While many of the changes associated with aging are inevitable, a surprising number can be controlled or modified. Shown here are 14 specific aspects of the aging process that can be prevented or modified through changes in life-style.

WHAT TO DO

Concern about the relationship between life-style and health is not a recent phenomenon. For centuries, physicians have discussed and debated what constitutes a healthy life-style. Today we have a better understanding of what is healthy and what is not than at any previous time in human history. There is, we now know, a clear relationship between the way in which we live and our health. And we know too that how we live in our earlier years can often affect our health and vitality in our later ones. Here then are some practical steps you can take to increase your chances for aging in a healthful manner. Each suggestion is accompanied by a brief discussion of its specific benefits.

Exercise Regularly

Exercise improves both mental and physical health. It increases resistance to disease and provides a healthy outlet for stress. [4]

(continued on p. 114)

Helen Glashow is working out on a treadmill, panting faintly, her brow furrowed in concentration. A red digital readout on the treadmill control panel registers 2.5 miles per hour. She will keep this up for 30 minutes or so, a routine she usually follows four times a week.

Similar scenes can be found in most any health club. What makes this one remarkable is that Glashow is 85 years old, the "health club" she is using is a converted dining room of the Hebrew Home for the Aged at Riverdale in the Bronx, and before she began her workouts last year she walked with a cane because of phlebitis and sciatica.

Elderly Enjoying Benefits of Exercise

As the treadmill motor whirls and her walking shoes slap the belt, the cane is nowhere to be seen.

For many years as the exercise boom swept the country, the elderly were ignored where workouts, cardiovascular fitness and building muscle mass were concerned. But in recent years, research has begun to show that the elderly who exercise can increase their strength and muscle mass, that their cardiovascular system will respond to exercise just as a younger person's will, that joints can become less stiff.

This has led some nursing homes to begin to introduce fitness classes. The Hebrew Home opened such a center last year and the residents who regularly attend the classes report that they feel better over all, are less stiff and find the activities enjoyable.

As often happens when fitness programs are introduced into institutional settings, the impetus comes from someone high in management. In this case it was Jacob Reingold, the home's executive vice president, who is an active runner at age 74. When told three decades ago that he needed knee surgery, Reingold shopped around until he found an orthopedist who suggested exercise instead.

"I have a very personal belief in exercise," he said, explaining why he pushed for what the home calls a "wellness center."

"These people tell me they feel better, their appetite is better, they sleep better, they can walk better," he said.

Response from residents here has borne out his belief about the benefits of exercise for the elderly.

"I feel more active, I can walk and move around better," said Clara Simon, 85, after one exercise class last week. Sue Shapiro, 78, also reported more ease of movement, and Joseph Kornbluh, 93, said, leaning on his cane after the session, "It keeps you from being so lazy."

Charles Bronz, the Hebrew Home's fitness coordinator who has a master's degree in physical education, uses armchairs as the center of the workouts.

The participants begin by sitting and performing arm and leg stretches, followed by modified situps in which they slouch down in their chairs and then lean forward. They hold elastic streamers in both hands and pass them under their feet or thighs and pull against the resistance to strengthen muscles. They stand and hold the back of the chairs and do modest leg raises. Bronz's aim is to strengthen wrists, ankles, quadriceps, abdominal and hip flexor muscles.

One goal is to increase the length of an individual's stride. Anyone whose stride is under 16 inches is considered in danger of a bad fall that could lead to a broken hip, which often precipitates an irreversible decline in health. Bronz wants to get the stride length up to over 24 inches, considered low risk.

The arm waving and resistance movements can increase heart rate slightly, leading over several months to a cardiovascular training effect. Bronz said some patients who entered the program with heart rates in the 100 range, considered high, had brought them down to a normal 70's range. Bronz thinks that increased cardiovascular fitness increases the amount of oxygen in the blood, which in turn increases oxygen reaching the brain.

"I think they feel better because of this," he said.

But Reingold and Bronz agree that the positive effects they ascribe are anecdotal, difficult to prove. It is possible that the residents feel better because they have been told they should feel better. Pinning down the claim that the exercise has lowered the residents' heart rates would require a sophisticated study in which one group that exercised was compared with another that did not.

"I think it costs less to care for the fit old, and I would like to do a study to prove that," Reingold said. "But we lack the funding for such research."

In a society that is often results-oriented, administrators like Reingold must worry about proving the efficacy of what they advocate. He must justify the money he has spent, prove that his program is beneficial if he wants to raise more money, whether for research or more staff, both goals he has.

Glashow is oblivious to this. She takes up her station on the treadmill because, she said: "You need something to do. Your mind needs to be occupied."

In terms of mobility at least, it appears to have significantly transformed her life. Most importantly, she has learned a basic lesson about fitness: it should be enjoyable.

So last week after the class had ended and the others filed from the room, there she was on the treadmill, zipping along under Bronz's watchful eye.

Source: William Stockton, *New York Times*, 12 June 1989, C11.

Did You Know That . . .

Studies have shown that older people who exercise can significantly improve their strength and endurance. For example, after President Reagan was shot in 1980, his doctors put him on a weight-lifting regimen. In the year that followed, he increased the size of his chest by three inches, a marked improvement in a man of 70.

Fluid intelligence: The ability to solve new or novel problems not previously encountered; reasoning power; often contrasted with *crystallized intelligence*, the ability to apply lessons from past experience to familiar situations or problems.

As a result, those who exercise regularly outlive their more sedentary peers. [5] In addition, according to Albert Rosenfeld, evidence "suggests that exercise can hold off many of the functional failings of aging [such as] the loss of bone strength and muscle mass, for example. Overall energy, stamina, agility, aerobic and cardiac capacity remain higher in exercisers than in the sedentary; the same advantage seems to hold for healthy levels of blood pressure, sugar, and cholesterol, not to mention mental outlook. Just about every study . . . shows that hardy oldsters . . . remain physically active all their lives." [6]

Furthermore, because exercise is so stimulating, it often helps sustain our ability to make decisions spontaneously, an ability known as **fluid intelligence**. Insel and Roth note that "exercise is the closest thing we have to a magic anti-aging pill and the fountain of youth: it slows the aging process and lessens the chances of disease." [7]

FIGURE 6.1
A Menu of Health-Saving Tactics

✔✔✔ Highly effective   ✔✔ Moderately effective   ✔ Somewhat effective

	No tobacco	Low-fat diet	High-fiber diet	Avoid alcohol	Avoid salted, pickled foods	Diet high in vegetables and fruits	Exercise, weight control
Cancer							
Lung	✔✔✔	✔				✔	
Breast		✔✔	✔			✔✔	✔
Colon		✔✔✔	✔✔✔			✔✔✔	✔
Liver				✔✔✔	✔	✔✔	
Heart attack	✔✔✔	✔✔✔				✔✔	✔✔
Stroke	✔				✔✔✔	✔✔	✔✔
Adult diabetes		✔✔✔	✔			✔✔	✔✔

Source: American Health Foundation.

The American Health Foundation has ranked the values of various dietary habits that may reduce the risk of developing a particular disease. Although healthful habits are not a guarantee against disease, this chart does indicate that a diet high in fruits and vegetables and low in fat has the highest protective effect.

Eat Right

There is little evidence that diet alone determines life expectancy. [8] However, in conjunction with other aspects of a healthy lifestyle, eating properly can increase your life span by as much as 6 to 10 years. [9] As Figure 6.1 suggests, diet can help prevent many of the chronic diseases associated with old age, including various cancers, heart disease, stroke, and diabetes. [10] Finally, eating wisely will help you maintain a desirable weight.

Maintain Your Normal Weight

According to one source, "Obesity actually produces premature aging. The fat person deteriorates in the same way as the slim person, only earlier." [11] Staying trim reduces your risk of suffering high blood pressure, strokes, gallstones, and liver diseases. [12] For further information on the importance of weight control and some practical suggestions on how to do it, see the volume in this series entitled *Wellness: Weight Control.*

Don't Smoke

Most people know that cigarette smoking has been linked specifically with lung cancer and heart disease. As you saw earlier, these highly preventable conditions are among the major causes of premature death. Studies have also found that smoking has "widespread deleterious effects on cardiovascular functioning, the respiratory system, and taste and smell perceptions." [13] The effects of tobacco use are more fully described in *Wellness: Tobacco & Health*, another volume in this series.

Drink Moderately, If at All

Heavy alcohol consumption can damage various organs of the body, particularly the brain and the liver. You may be surprised to learn that some experts assert that more than one drink a day for women, or 2 drinks a day for men, is excessive. And as age takes its toll on vision, hearing, and reflex speed, the dulling effects of alcohol consumption can only aggravate preexisting conditions. Finally, alcohol is a leading cause of fatal automobile accidents; it can instantaneously extinguish a life, regardless of age. For more information on this important topic, see *Wellness: Alcohol, Use & Abuse,* in this series.

Adopt a Positive Mental Attitude

If your attitude toward aging is positive and healthy, the process and the changes associated with it are not likely to interfere with your ability to engage in and enjoy life's activities. "Your attitude in sickness and in health is extremely important in determining

Did You Know That . . .

Many experts believe that if you feel good about your yourself, especially about your health, you are likely to live longer than someone who is pessimistic. A recent study of 100-year-olds by the National Institute of Aging found that every one of them shared positive attitudes toward life. All still made plans for future events and looked forward to special occasions.

FIGURE 6.2
Nutrition and Aging

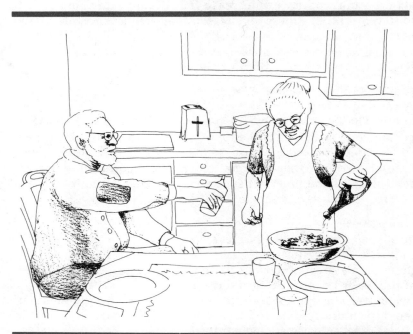

Nutritional and caloric needs change as a person ages. It is important to eat healthy foods, such as salads of fresh vegetables, and also to match the amount of food consumed to one's caloric needs.

the quality and duration of life." [14] In fact, thinking young may help you remain young in spirit, and that may, in turn, actually retard the biological processes of aging. In 1979, Norman Cousins, then an adjunct professor in the School of Medicine at the University of California at Los Angeles, observed, "One of the most important things in life is the need not to accept downside predictions from experts. . . . No one knows enough to make a pronouncement of doom." [15]

Your beliefs about old age can further affect your physical and psychological well-being as you age. The holistic health advisers Gordon Edlin and Eric Golanty assert that "If you believe that infirmity and senility are the inevitable consequences of old age, your mind has the power to produce the destructive changes in physiology that lead to these afflictions.

(continued on p. 118)

The Best Is Yet to Come

Leo Tolstoy, who completed his novel *Anna Karenina* at the age of 49, took his first bike-riding lesson at the age of 67. We seldom think of old age as a time for major accomplishments, but as the list below proves, old age in no way signals the decline of a person's potential.

60—After nearly 15 years of lobbying by British feminist Emmeline Pankhurst, her "Representation of the People Act" passes in 1918, giving women the right to vote.

61—John Adams becomes President (1796–1800), as does Andrew Jackson (1828–1836).

62—Louis Pasteur administers the first vaccine against rabies.

63—J.R.R. Tolkien publishes the third and last volume of *The Fellowship of the Ring*. He had written *The Hobbit* at 45.

64—Oscar Hammerstein II writes the lyrics for *The Sound of Music*.

65—Douglas MacArthur is appointed the effective ruler and "Shogun" of Japan during its occupation at the conclusion of World War II.

66—Michelangelo completes the "Last Judgment" on the altar wall of the Sistine Chapel, Rome.

67—Sigmund Freud writes *The Ego and the Id*.

68—Lillian Carter (mother of Jimmy) joins the Peace Corps and spends the next 2 years working as a nurse at a clinic near Bombay, India.

69—Elihu Yale sends books and other gifts to a new college and the college then calls itself "Yale."

70—Friedrich Engels continues to read seven daily newspapers, in three languages; and he reads nineteen weeklies, in eight languages.

71—Coco Chanel invents the Chanel suit and emerges as a major force in the fashion world.

72—Charles Darwin publishes his last book, the topic of which is earthworms.

73—Peter Mark Roget completes *Roget's Thesaurus*.

74—Frank Lloyd Wright makes his first drawings of the Guggenheim Museum, New York City.

75—Henry Ford is still fit enough to do handstands; he gets into convertibles by leaping over the door.

76—H. G. Wells completes his doctoral dissertation and receives the D. Sc. from London University. He had left school at 14.

Did You Know That . . .

One of the positive aspects of aging is the experience and wisdom we can gain. As we age, we learn more about ourselves and others. In the process, we develop a greater sense of self-confidence and become better able to handle daily stress.

77—Claude Monet begins work on a complete room of paintings of water lilies. They become the "Sistine Chapel of Impressionism."

78—Matisse designs the Chapel of the Rosary, Vence, France.

79—Voltaire is told by his doctor that coffee is a poison; but he replies "I've been poisoning myself for 80 years."

80—Grandma Moses has her first solo show, and goes on to paint for another 20 years.

Source: Adapted from Jeremy Baker, *Tolstoy's Bicycle* (New York: St. Martin's Press, 1982).

Mental depression, negative attitudes, and a loss of interest in life will lower immunological defenses, reduce vitality, and increase the likelihood of disease and incapacitating illness." [16] What you think can become so.

Recognize and Reduce Stress

As one humorist observed, "Death is nature's way of telling you to slow down." There are a number of steps you can take to reduce the pressure and stress caused by everyday life. Walk or bicycle to work or school. Make recreation a regular part of your activities. Make and keep friends of all ages. Allow time for rest and relaxation and get adequate sleep daily. Pursue work that you find satisfying or strive to find satisfaction in the work you do.

Consult appropriate health-care professionals: Regular visits to your physician, eye doctor, and dentist will help them detect any early signs of aging that require attention. A number of specialized health-care professionals are concerned specifically with aging. Their field of study, **geriatrics**, is devoted to care for the aging, including the problems and diseases of older adults. **Gerontology** is the branch of science dealing with the aging process. Experts in this field are called gerontologists, who study the phenomena and problems of aging and are concerned with all its aspects, including its biological, medical, social, and psychological ramifications.

Take stock of your mental and physical health habits. Now is the best time to adopt the needed attitudes, strategies, and practices that will allow you to maintain the best mind and body possible when you reach your 60s, 70s, and 80s. Today, while you have control over most changes that will occur as you age, what

Geriatrics: The branch of medicine concerned with the care and treatment of elders.

Gerontology: The branch of science concerned with the study of the aging process, including its biological, psychological, social, and health-related aspects.

FIGURE 6.3
Stress Test

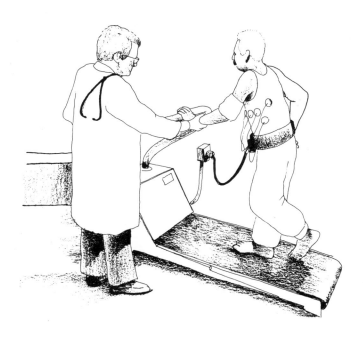

Periodic physical exams are a useful tool for monitoring your health, detecting early warning signs of certain diseases, and planning life-style changes. Depending on your medical history and condition, your physician may, for example, recommend that you take a stress test before beginning a new exercise program.

you do *to* and *for* yourself now can prolong your health and vigor—and keep them as vital a part of your future life as they are at your present age.

A PLAN FOR ACTION

We've said it before, and we'll say it again: Every individual has a powerful influence upon the quality and rate of his or her own aging process. Good health at every stage in your life cycle is a worthwhile goal in its own right. A life-style that promotes good health will, among many other benefits, help prevent the premature onset of chronic disease and will minimize the impact of those conditions that do occur.

Commitment Form for a Healthy Life-Style

I, _____ _____, have decided that I need to _____ in order to increase my life expectancy. I promise to begin my _____ program below starting on _____, 19____, and to continue with it until _____ (a date not more than three months from now).

My program for more healthy behavior is:

1. _____

_____

_____

_____

2. _____

_____

_____

_____

3. _____

_____

_____

_____

Signed: _____ Date: _____

Witness: _____ Date: _____

Implementing the steps called for here and in chapters 3 and 5 requires both a plan of action and a self-management program. Your plan can consist of 3 steps. First, commit to making the appropriate changes in your life-style as called for above. The commitment form on page 120 can help you make and keep the promises essential to healthful aging.

Second, monitor your progress. Keep a written record of your goals and the actions you take to achieve them on a daily or weekly basis. Try to come up with a method of keeping track numerically of your progress—the number of fast-food or unhealthy meals you cut back on, the number of pounds lost, or the number of miles walked or jogged. Set realistic weekly goals and reward yourself when you meet them.

Third, evaluate the system you have set up and are following for any behavior that still leads you astray of your goals. There may be some behaviors that you did not initially recognize as problem areas that now need to be addressed in order for you to meet your goals. Modify any practices that contribute to behaviors you want to change; also, plan necessary strategies that will maintain the positive changes you have brought about. Implement those strategies that will ensure that you *remain* changed.

If you take these steps, you are exponentially increasing your chances of leading not only a long life but a healthy, active one as well. As the gerontologist Ken Dychtwald notes, engaging in healthy practices can help us enjoy "an elongation of the periods of life we appreciate most—extra years of youthful adventure, a slowed-down middle age, a lengthened late adulthood, and a vigorous old age." [17] That is what we all wish for—and contrary to myths of aging, that is well within easy reach. W

Glossary

A

Absolute human life span: The maximum possible chronological age attainable by humans under ideal circumstances.

Acute disease: Any disease or illness whose onset is more or less sudden; acute diseases have a limited, usually brief, period of duration and vary greatly in severity.

Aging: The third and final stage of the life cycle, characterized by a continuation of learning, accompanied by a decline—at varying rates—in physical and mental skills and abilities.

Aging process: The ongoing series of regular and generally predictable changes in physical and mental condition that accompany an increase in chronological age.

Alkaline-based soaps: Soaps to which alkaline substances such as phosphates, carbonates, and silicates have been added in order to improve their cleaning ability in water that is acidic or contains a relatively heavy concentration of minerals (hard water).

Alzheimer's disease: An incurable organic disorder of the brain in which there is progressive loss of memory and other intellectual functions.

Atherosclerosis: A narrowing of the arteries caused by the buildup of fatty deposits (plaque) on the interior walls of the arteries.

Atrophy: A wasting away or progressive decline; degeneration.

Autoimmune reaction: A disorder in which the immune system attacks healthy tissue or a healthy organ or group of cells that it has mistakenly identified as a harmful, foreign invader.

B

Biological age: A person's age as determined by his or her overall physiological condition, expressed as the chronological age for which that condition is regarded as typical or average.

C

Cerebral atherosclerosis: A narrowing of the cerebral arteries caused by the gradual accumulation of fatty deposits (plaques) on the artery walls that reduces or blocks the flow of blood to portions of the brain.

Cerebral cortex: The outermost layer of the upper and largest portion of the brain (the cerebrum) that controls the higher cognitive functions, such as memory, speech, and thought.

Cholesterol: A fatlike substance found in animal foods and also manufactured by the body. Cholesterol is essential to nerve and brain cell function and to the synthesis of sex hormones, and is also a component of bile acids used to aid fat digestion. It is also a part of plaques that accumulate on artery walls in atherosclerosis.

Chronic disease: Any disease or illness that persists over an extended period of time, in contrast to acute diseases.

Chronological age: The actual length of time that a person has lived, usually measured in years.

Cognitive functioning: The capacity to perform the higher-order mental processes, such as perceiving, thinking, and knowing.

D

Dendrites: The branching structures of a nerve cell (neuron) that receive impulses from other nearby nerve cells.

Depression: A mental state, characterized by extreme sadness or dejection, that persists for an extended period of time.

DNA (deoxyribonucleic acid): The extraordinarily complex double helix–shaped molecule, found in the nucleus of cells and in viruses, that stores the genetic code.

E

Endocrine glands: Those glands in the body that secrete chemical substances called hormones (or endocrines) directly into the bloodstream to regulate vital bodily functions and processes; the pancreas, adrenal glands, thyroid, pituitary, ovaries, and testicles are all endocrine glands.

F

Fluid intelligence: The ability to solve new or novel problems not previously encountered; reasoning power; often contrasted with *crystallized intelligence*, the ability to apply lessons from past experience to familiar situations or problems.

Functional disorder: A mental or emotional disorder that cannot be associated with a known physical cause.

G

Geriatrics: The branch of medicine concerned with the care and treatment of elders.

Gerontology: The branch of science concerned with the study of the aging process, including its biological, psychological, social, and health-related aspects.

H

Homeostasis: The process by which the body regulates temperature, oxygen level, sugar content, and related factors necessary to optimum functioning in order to maintain them at constant levels.

Hormone: Any of the chemical substances, such as estrogen, that are released directly into the bloodstream by the endocrine glands and elicit specific responses from a targeted muscle, organ, or other bodily structure.

I

Immune system: The body's natural defense system, which works to eliminate pathogens.

L

Life expectancy: The estimated number of years of life remaining to a given individual at a given point in his or her life span.

Life span: The interval between birth and death which may be divided into 3 more or less distinct phases—maturation, maturity, and aging.

Lymphocytes: The specialized white blood cells that collectively identify, attack, and destroy harmful pathogens that invade the body; lymphocytes (white blood cells) are a crucial component of the immune system.

M

Maturation: The first stage of the life cycle, during which physical growth is completed, much learning takes place, and physical and mental abilities and skills reach their peak stage of development.

Maturity: The second stage of the life cycle, during which learning continues and physical and mental skills and abilities are maintained at a peak or near-peak stage of development.

Mean human life span: The chronological age by which 50 percent of a given human population will have died, according to statistical projections.

Menopause: The cessation of menstruation in the female, typically between the ages of 45 and 50.

Mental age: A person's level of intellectual functioning regardless of his or her chronological age; generally attributed to the French psychologist Alfred Binet (1857–1911).

Metabolize: To transform food into energy by breaking down large molecules into smaller ones, releasing energy in the process; the general process by which the body performs this function is known as the *metabolic process* or *metabolism*.

Mutation: An alteration in the structure of the DNA molecule that affects the functioning or structure of the larger organism; mutations may arise from a variety of causes, including environmental factors (radiation, exposure to chemicals) and random error during the cell division process; their effects may be either beneficial or harmful.

N

Neurons: The impulse-conducting cells that are the basic functioning units of the nervous system.

O

Organic disorder: A mental or emotional disorder that results from an identifiable physical cause.

Osteoporosis: A disturbance of bone metabolism in which the bone mass decreases and the bones become increasingly fragile.

P

Perception: The process by which a living organism comes to know or experience external objects and events on the basis of information reported by the sensory organs.

Pharmacology: The branch of medicine concerned with the discovery and development of drugs used in the treatment of disease.

Presbyopia: A condition in which the eye, as a result of normal aging, loses the elasticity necessary to focus on and clearly distinguish nearby objects; presbyopia normally first appears between ages 40 and 45 and can be remedied with reading glasses.

Psychomotor performance: The ability to react appropriately and in a timely manner to any stimulus that requires a coordinated physical (motor) and psychological response.

S

Scoliosis: Abnormal curvature of the spine to one side of the body; scoliosis occurs most frequently in children and adolescents, but may also affect adults.

Senile dementia: Any chronic organic mental disorder that is characterized by a gradual and irreversible deterioration of mental functions.

Senses: A living organism's physical means of detecting changes in the environment; humans have at least 10 senses, including vision, hearing, taste, smell, touch, pain, warmth, cold, equilibrium, and kinesthesis (the ability to sense the position and movement of the body and its various parts).

Sensory threshold: The minimum intensity or level of stimulation that a sensory organ must receive before it will transmit information about the stimulus to the brain.

Serum cholesterol: Cholesterol found in the clear fluid (serum) that separates from the blood when it clots.

Stress: Any external stimulus, whether physical or psychological, that necessitates resistance, change, or adaptation by the individual.

U

Ultraviolet rays: Light rays whose wavelength is less than that of the shortest visible light yet longer than that of X rays; prolonged exposure to ultraviolet light is potentially harmful.

V

Vital capacity: The maximum volume of air that can be expelled from the lungs after inhaling to one's maximum capacity, usually expressed as a ratio (volume of air out divided by volume of air in).

Notes

CHAPTER 1

1. John W. Wright, ed., *The Universal Almanac 1990* (New York: Andrews and McMeel, 1989), 225.
2. *The 1989 Information Please Almanac,* 42d ed. (Boston: Houghton Mifflin Co., 1988), 794.
3. Tom Biracree and Nancy Biracree, *Almanac of the American People* (New York: Facts On File, 1988), 6.
4. Adella J. Harris and Jonathan F. Feinberg, "Television and Aging: Is What You See What You Get?" *The Gerontologist* 17 (November 1977): 468.
5. *A Profile of Older Americans* (Washington, DC: American Association of Retired Persons, 1988), 3.
6. Compiled from a variety of sources including the following: American Association of Retired Persons, *Truth About Aging* (Washington, DC: American Association of Retired Persons, 1984), 12; Geri Marr Burdman, *Healthful Aging* (Englewood Cliffs, NJ: Prentice-Hall, 1986), 13; Benjamin F. Miller, M.D., and Claire Brackman Keane, R.N., B.S., M.Ed., *Encyclopedia and Dictionary of Medicine, Nursing, and Allied Health*, 3d edition (Philadelphia: W. B. Saunders Co., 1983), 27; and National Institute on Aging, *What Is Your Aging IQ?* (November 1986): 1–2.
7. "85 Seen as Average Life Span," *Centre Daily Times,* 2 November 1990, 5A.
8. Armeda F. Ferrini and Rebecca L. Ferrini, *Health in the Later Years* (Dubuque, IA: William C. Brown Co., 1989), 350.
9. Paul M. Insel and Walton T. Roth, *Core Concepts in Health* (Mountain View, CA: Mayfield Publishing Co., 1988), 529.

CHAPTER 2

1. James E. Birren and J. V. Renner, "Research on the Psychology of Aging," in *Handbook of the Psychology of Aging,* James E. Birren and K. Warner Schaie, eds. (New York: Van Nostrand Reinhold, 1977), 4.
2. Biracree and Biracree, p. 8.
3. Robert C. Atchley, *Social Forces and Aging,* 5th ed. (Belmont, CA: Wadsworth Publishing Co., 1988), 70.

4. Gordon Edlin and Eric Golanty, *Health and Wellness: A Holistic Approach,* 3d ed. (Boston: Jones & Bartlett, 1988), 483.

5. Leonard Hayflick, "The Cell Biology of Human Aging," *New England Journal of Medicine* (2 December 1976): 1302.

6. Insel and Roth, p. 527.

7. Daniel Rudman et al., "Effects of Human Growth Hormone in Men Over 60 Years Old," *New England Journal of Medicine* 323:1 (5 July 1990): 1.

8. Jodie DeJonge, "Man Doesn't Regret Flirtation with 'Fountain of Youth,'" *Centre Daily Times,* 11 November 1990, C1.

9. Bernard L. Strehler, "A New Age for Aging," *Natural History* (February 1973), 343.

10. K. Warner Schaie and Sherry L. Willis, *Adult Development and Aging,* 2d ed. (Boston: Little, Brown & Co., 1986), 372.

11. Insel and Roth, p. 527.

12. Edlin and Golanty, p. 486.

13. Burdman, p. 24.

14. Atchley, p. 71.

15. Atchley, p. 71.

16. Nathan W. Shock, "System Integration," in *Handbook of the Biology of Aging,* Caleb E. Finch and Leonard Hayflick, eds. (New York: Van Nostrand Reinhold, 1977), 639–665.

17. Insel and Roth, p. 526.

18. David Gelman, "Why We Age Differently," *Newsweek,* 20 October 1986, 61.

19. Gelman, p. 61.

20. Bernard L. Strehler, *Time, Cells, and Aging* (New York: Academic Press, 1977), 12–116.

21. Shock, pp. 639–665.

22. Edlin and Golanty, p. 482.

23. Elsworth R. Buskirk, "Health Maintenance and Longevity: Exercise," in *Handbook of the Biology of Aging,* 2d ed., Caleb E. Finch and Leonard Hayflick, eds. (New York: Van Nostrand Reinhold, 1985), 894–931.

24. Susan K. Whitbourne, *The Aging Body: Physiological Changes and Psychological Consequences* (New York: Springer-Verlag, 1985), 21.

25. Insel and Roth, p. 516.

26. Insel and Roth, p. 516.

27. Jane F. Desforges, ed., "Current Concepts," *New England Journal of Medicine* 322:20 (17 May 1990): 1441.

28. Jody W. Zylke, "As Nation Grows Older, Falls Become Greater Source of Fear, Injury, Death," *Journal of the American Medical Association* 263:15 (18 April 1990): 2021.

29. "The Exercise Elixir," *American Health* (July/August 1989): 68.
30. Atchley, p. 73.
31. Atchley, p. 74.
32. William H. Lee, "The Birth of a Wrinkle," *Health News & Review* (September/October 1989): 5.
33. Bernice L. Neugarten et al., "Women's Attitudes Toward the Menopause," *Vita Humana* 6:140.
34. Insel and Roth, p. 516.

CHAPTER 3

1. Robert C. Atchley, *Social Forces and Aging,* 4th ed. (Belmont, CA: Wadsworth Publishing Co., 1985), 75.
2. Atchley, 4th ed., p. 76.
3. *A Profile of Older Americans* (Washington, DC: American Association of Retired Persons, 1988), 13.
4. Special Committee of the United States Senate on Aging *Aging America: Trends and Projections* No. 101-J (Washington, DC: Government Printing Office, 1990), 81–82.
5. Insel and Roth, p. 516.
6. Whitbourne, p. 2.
7. Burdman, p. 38.

CHAPTER 4

1. Roy L. Walford, *Maximum Life Span* (New York: W. W. Norton & Co., 1983), 59.
2. Edlin and Golanty, p. 487.
3. Insel and Roth, p. 517.
4. Albert Rosenfeld, *Prolongevity II* (New York: Alfred A. Knopf, 1985), 179.
5. Caroline Hall Otis, "Pumping Intellect," *Utne Reader* (January/February 1989): 32.
6. Atchley, 5th ed., p. 83.
7. Ferrini and Ferrini, p. 88.
8. Insel and Roth, p. 517.
9. Atchley, 5th ed., p. 87.
10. Burdman, p. 27.
11. Atchley, 5th ed., p. 88.
12. Atchley, 5th ed., p. 88.
13. Atchley, 5th ed., pp. 89–90.

14. A. T. Welford, "Sensory, Perceptual, and Motor Processes in Older Adults," *Handbook of Mental Health and Aging,* James E. Birren and R. Bruce Sloane, eds. (Englewood Cliffs, NJ: Prentice-Hall, 1980), 205.

15. *Older & Wiser: The Baltimore Longitudinal Study of Aging,* National Institutes of Mental Health (September 1989), 36.

16. *Older & Wiser,* p. 37.

17. Schaie and Willis, p. 337.

18. Atchley, 5th ed., pp. 91–96.

19. A. E. David Schoenfield, "Learning, Memory, and Aging," in *Handbook of Mental Health and Aging,* James E. Birren and R. Bruce Sloane, eds. (Englewood Cliffs, NJ: Prentice-Hall, 1980), 240.

20. Schaie and Willis, p. 337.

CHAPTER 5

1. *Coping With Growing Older* (Alexandria, VA: National Mental Health Association), 1.

2. Atchley, 4th ed., p. 108.

3. Atchley, 4th ed., p. 109.

4. Ruth Kay, *Plain Talk About Aging* (Washington, DC: National Institutes of Mental Health, 1985), 2.

5. Beni Habot and Leslie S. Libow, "The Interrelationship of Mental and Physical Status and Its Assessment in the Older Adult: Mind-Body Interaction," in *Handbook of Mental Health and Aging,* Birren and Sloane, eds.

6. Atchley, 4th ed., p. 108.

7. "Alzheimer's Disease: Mystery of the Mind," *FDA Consumer* (September 1989), 19.

8. Rosenfeld, p. 227.

9. Insel and Roth, p. 528.

10. Rosenfeld, p. 231.

11. Walford, p. 59.

12. Robert A. Wiswell, "Relaxation, Exercise, and Aging," in *Handbook of Mental Health and Aging,* Birren and Sloane, eds., p. 955.

13. Edlin and Golanty, p. 489.

14. Charles M. Gaitz and Roy V. Varner, "Preventive Aspects of Mental Illness in Late Life," in *Handbook of Mental Health and Aging,* Birren and Sloane, eds., p. 969.

15. Rosenfeld, p. 180.

CHAPTER 6

1. Insel and Roth, p. 516.
2. Insel and Roth, p. 517.
3. Edlin and Golanty, p. 486.
4. Isadore Rosenfeld, *Modern Prevention: The New Medicine* (New York: Simon & Schuster, 1986), 68.
5. Rebecca J. Donatelle et al., *Access to Health* (Englewood Cliffs, NJ: Prentice-Hall, 1988), 434.
6. A. Rosenfeld, p. 228.
7. Insel and Roth, p. 519.
8. Donatelle, p. 434.
9. Donatelle, p. 434.
10. I. Rosenfeld, p. 69.
11. Insel/Roth, p. 519.
12. Edward L. Bortz, *Creative Aging* (New York: Macmillan, 1963), 140.
13. Whitbourne, p. 226.
14. I. Rosenfeld, p. 70.
15. "Beyond Positive Thinking," *Success* (December 1988), 32.
16. Edlin and Golanty, p. 481.
17. Jean Dietz, "Life Span Lengthening," *Centre Daily Times,* 8 October 1990, C1.

Resources

BOOKS

Anderson, Bob. *Stretching*. New York: Random House, 1980.

This useful book shows the importance of stretching for fitness, tone, and muscle flexibility. More than 200 stretches and stretching routines for 36 different sports and activities are illustrated with more than 1,000 drawings.

Belsky, Janet K. *Here Tomorrow: Making the Most of Life After Fifty*. Baltimore: Johns Hopkins University Press, 1988.

The author notes that more Americans are living longer than ever before. Belsky shows that aging can be a positive experience and provides answers to questions about work and retirement, love and marriage, the death of a spouse, health and the aging body, hobbies, leisure, and more.

Berman, Phillip L., ed. *The Courage to Grow Old*. New York: Ballantine, 1989.

This book of essays by actors, scientists, economists, and teachers shows that old age can be the most creative, fulfilling period in a person's life, rather than a time of decline. The book is inspiring and uplifting.

Burstein, Nancy. *Soft Aerobics: The New Low-Impact Workout*. New York: Putnam, 1987.

This book presents an alternative to traditional, high-impact aerobics (which can cause injury from excess stress on ankles, shins, calves, knees, hips, and back). Twelve low-impact exercises combined into 4 distinct exercise routines are presented and illustrated with step-by-step photographs. Readers can follow the specific routines presented in the book or create a personalized program for individual fitness levels. The program is effective for maintaining fitness, losing weight, and preventing osteoporosis in women.

Callahan, Daniel. *Setting Limits: Medical Goals in an Aging Society*. New York: Simon & Schuster, 1987.

Callahan tackles the ethical questions of extending the lives of the elderly and shows that the American health-care system gives little thought to the quality of these extended lives. The author maintains that medicine has had the specific goal of averting premature death but should shift attention to the relief of suffering rather than merely to extending life.

Carlin, Vivian F., and Ruth Mansberg. *If I Live to Be 100: Congregate Housing for Later Life*. West Nyack, New York: Parker Publishing, 1984.

This guide shows how to select the right housing situation for retirement, based on individual retirement needs for such factors as new friends and acquaintances, security, community planning or hobby groups, or access to a staffed medical clinic or nursing care facility. The author presents interviews with residents living in a congregate housing situation who explain their reasons for choosing this type of retirement housing and discuss their adjustments to apartment living.

Egginton, Mary, Maryann Kunigonis, Joan Mintz, and Dorothy Roser. *An Older Woman's Health Guide*. New York: McGraw-Hill, 1984.

The authors present information to dispel negative views of older women, including the stereotypes that older women are physically unattractive or a burden to grown children. The book includes a careful analysis of social and family relationships, various educational and employment opportunities, legal resources, money management, and, most importantly, health care.

Ferrini, Armeda F., and Rebecca L. Ferrini. *Health in the Later Years*. Dubuque, IA: William C. Brown Publishers, 1989.

This comprehensive book provides an overview of health and aging. It presents basic health principles as they apply to personal health in the elderly and discusses health-related issues of concern to older citizens and those who work with them. Topics include a description of elderly persons and discussions of biological aging, changes that occur with aging, chronic and acute illness, nutrition, physical activity, sexuality, medical care, long-term care, dying, death, and grieving.

Fries, James F., M.D. *Aging Well: A Guide for Successful Seniors*. New York: Addison-Wesley, 1989.

Dr. Fries offers advice and information on growing older in good health and good spirits. The book addresses issues of maintaining vitality, self-care for common medical problems, diet and exercise, sexuality and aging, living with chronic medical ailments, and retirement and financial planning.

Halpern, James. *Helping Your Aging Parents: A Practical Guide for Adult Children*. New York: McGraw-Hill, 1987.

This book is for those children of aging parents who find that they must struggle with the burden of contemplating their parents' future while maintaining their own families and careers. Halpern offers constructive advice and support on both the practical and emotional aspects of caring for elderly parents.

Kaplan, Lawrence J. *Retiring Right: Planning for Your Successful Retirement*. Wayne, NJ: Avery Publishing Group, 1987.

A guide to help plan a financially secure and fulfilling retirement. The author answers questions about savings and investment income, tax shelters, Social Security, and private benefits. Advice is also provided about insurance, estate planning, housing options, and what to do with free time once retired. The book includes personalized guides and worksheets.

Langholz, Edna et al., *The Nutrition Game: The Right Moves If You're Over 50*. San Leandro, CA: Bristol Publishing Enterprises, 1990.

The authors discuss many nutrition issues, dispel old myths, and present information for people wishing to modify their diets to reduce fat, increase fiber, and attain better health.

Meyers, Casey. *Aerobic Walking: The Best and Safest Weight Loss and Cardiovascular Exercise for Everyone Overweight or Out of Shape*. New York: Random House, 1987.

This book addresses the benefits of walking for the purpose of disease prevention and helping with weight-control problems. Covered are the proper walking gaits for maximum aerobic benefits and reduced stress on joints and how to develop a self-tailored fitness walking program.

Miller, Sigmund Stephen, Julian Asher Miller, and Don Ethan Miller. *Conquest of Aging: The Definitive Home Medical Reference from a Panel of Distinguished Medical Authorities*. New York: Macmillan, 1986.

The authors demonstrate that the usual decline in health, vitality, and memory associated with growing older is neither inevitable nor insurmountable. Well-being can be maintained through a sensible combination of exercise, diet, and proper use of prescription and over-the-counter medications.

Skala, Ken. *American Guidance for Those Over 60*. Falls Church, VA: American Guidance, Inc., 1990.

A guidebook of benefits, entitlements, and available assistance for senior Americans. The book tells how the U.S. government and the nation's people provide programs to help older Americans with currently available resources. Topics covered include Medicare and Medicaid, housing, nursing homes and home care, pharmaceuticals, funerals, Social Security, supplemental income, health and health insurance, food stamps, legal and tax assistance, and more.

Vierck, Elizabeth. *Fact Book on Aging*. Santa Barbara, CA: ABC-CLIO, Inc., 1990.

The statistical profile of the average senior citizen is provided in this book. Facts are presented on the size and growth of the older population, work and retirement, income, housing, crime, religion, health, and other topics.

Wells, Joel. *Who Do You Think You Are? How to Build Self-Esteem*. Chicago, IL: Thomas More Press, 1989.

This book shows how to strengthen self-esteem by accepting one's self and taking pride in personal affairs. It includes chapters for senior citizens and the widowed and divorced. The book provides specific steps to take to build self-esteem.

NEWSLETTERS

AARP Bulletin is published by the American Association of Retired Persons and covers timely issues on health, fitness, results of lobby efforts before Congress, and other concerns of people over age 50. A one-year subscription costs $5, and this fee includes an annual subscription to *Modern Maturity* and a year-long membership in the AARP. Write AARP Membership Processing Center, P.O. Box 199, Long Beach, CA 90801.

ACSH News and Views is published 5 times a year by the American Council on Science and Health, a nonprofit educational association. The newsletter discusses topics related to food, chemicals, the environment, and health. A one-year subscription is $15. Write to ACSH News and Views, 1995 Broadway, New York, NY 10023, or call (212) 362-7044.

Consumer Reports Health Letter is published monthly by Consumers Union of the United States, a nonprofit organization that provides information and advice on goods, services, health, and personal finance. A one-year subscription is $24, and the cost for 2 years is $38. Write to the Subscription Director, Consumer Reports Health Letter, Box 56356, Boulder, CO 80322-6356, or call (800) 274-8370.

Harvard Health Letter is published monthly as a nonprofit service by the Department of Continuing Education, Harvard Medical School, in association with Harvard University Press. The letter has the goal of interpreting health information for general readers in a timely and accurate fashion. A one-year subscription is $21. Write to the Harvard Medical School Letter, 79 Garden Street, Cambridge, MA 02138, or call customer service at (617) 495-3975.

Healthline is published monthly by Healthline Publishing, Inc. The letter is intended to educate readers about ways to help themselves avoid illness and live longer, healthier lives. A one-year subscription is $19, or $34 for 2 years. Write to Healthline, The C. V. Mosby Company, 11830 Westline Industrial Drive, St. Louis, MO 63146-3318, or call (800) 325-4177 (ext. 351).

Johns Hopkins Medical Letter, Health After 50 is published monthly by Medletter Associates, Inc., and covers a variety of topics related to healthful living. A one-year subscription is $20. Write to the Johns Hopkins Medical Letter, P.O. Box 420179, Palm Coast, FL 32142.

Lahey Clinic Health Letter is published monthly to bring readers timely, relevant information about important medical issues. Continuing topics include general healthfulness, natural and processed foods, depression, exercise, alcohol, prescription medicine therapy, major diseases, and exercise. A one-year subscription is $18. Write to the Lahey Clinic Health Letter, Subscription Department, P.O. Box 541, Burlington, MA 01805.

Mayo Clinic Nutrition Letter is published monthly and provides reliable information about nutrition and fitness and how decisions on these matters affect your health. A one-year subscription is $24. Write to the Mayo Foundation for Medical Education and Research, 200 1st Street SW, Rochester, MN 55905, or call (800) 888-3968.

Tufts University Diet and Nutrition Letter is published monthly and covers nutrition and wellness, exercise, diet, disease, and food consumerism. A one-year subscription costs $20. Write to the Tufts University Diet and Nutrition Letter, 53 Park Place, New York, NY 10007.

University of California Berkeley Wellness Letter is published monthly and covers many topics, including nutrition, fitness, and stress management. A one-year subscription is $20. Write to the University of California, Berkeley Wellness Letter, P.O. Box 420148, Palm Coast, FL 32142.

PERIODICALS

American Health Magazine: Fitness of Body and Mind is published 10 times a year and covers various aspects of physical and mental well-being. In addition to feature articles, ongoing departments include Nutrition News, Fitness Reports, Mind/Body News, Family Report, Family Pet, and more. A one-year subscription is $14.95. Write to American Health: Fitness of Body and Mind, P.O. Box 3015, Harlan, IA 51537-3015.

Current Health 2: The Continuing Guide to Health Education is published monthly from September through May. Each issue contains a feature article plus a number of shorter pieces on topics such as drugs, psychology, your personal health, disease, and nutrition. For subscription information, contact *Current Health 2,* Publication and Subscription Offices, Field Publications, 4343 Equity Drive, Columbus, Ohio 43228.

In Health Magazine is published 6 times a year and provides articles on a number of health issues. In addition to recipes and practical nutrition tips, the magazine regularly includes self-help resources for consumers. A one-year subscription is $18. Write to In Health, P.O. Box 52431, Boulder, CO 80321-2431.

Modern Maturity is published bimonthly by the American Association of Retired Persons (AARP) and covers topics of health, health insurance, medicine, nutrition, finances, and more. Each issue also spotlights seniors on the move and presents feature articles on everything from job hunting after 50 to recipes to hiking through remote sections of the world. A one-year subscription costs $5 and includes the *AARP Bulletin* and a year-long membership in the AARP. Write AARP Membership Processing Center, P.O. Box 199, Long Beach, CA 90801.

Priorities: For Long Life & Good Health is published quarterly by the American Council of Science and Health, Inc. (ACSH), a nonprofit consumer education association concerned with nutrition, chemicals, life-style factors, the environment, and human health. General individual membership in ACSH, which includes a subscription to *Priorities,* costs $25 a year. Write to the Subscription Department, Priorities, 1995 Broadway, 16th Floor, New York, NY 10023-5860.

HOTLINES

Alzheimer's Disease and Related Disorders Association, (800) 621-0379. Offers assistance, referrals, and information to Alzheimer's families through its 188 chapters nationwide. The mailing address is P.O. Box 5675, Department PX1, Chicago, IL 60680.

National Council on Aging, (800) 424-9046, provides information for care-givers and, upon request, a publications catalog.

National Health Information Clearing House, Department of Health and Human Services, (800) 336-4797; in Maryland, call (301) 656-4167. Operated by the Office of Disease Prevention and Health Promotion, this information and referral center's trained personnel will direct callers to the organization or government agency that can assist with health questions, whether they are about high blood pressure, cancer, fitness, or any other topic. Available 9:00 A.M. to 5:00 P.M., eastern standard time, Monday through Friday.

Tel-Med is a free telephone service provided in many cities. Callers can ask for a specific tape number and have the health message played over the telephone. There are over 300 medical topics to choose from, including topics related to maintaining a healthy life-style. Many states provide toll-free numbers for this service. Call the local information operator to find the nearest Tel-Med office, or write to Tel-Med, Box 970, Colton, CA 92324.

VIDEOTAPES

The following video program can be ordered from the National Wellness Institute, Inc., South Hall, 1319 Fremont Street, Stevens Point, WI 54481.

Write for format, price, and ordering information.

Swing into Shape is a low-intensity nonaerobic exercise video for the aging population. It focuses on the improvement of muscle tone, strength, and flexibility. The 3 instructive 26-minute routines are designed to acknowledge the physical limitations of this population. The exercises were designed by Betsy Bork, a physical therapist.

The next 3 videos are available from Nutrition Counseling and Education Services (NC&ES), P.O. Box 3018, Olathe, KS 66062-3018. Write for prices and ordering information or call (913) 782-8230. The following toll-free number is for placing orders only, (800) 445-5653. All videos in VHS format only.

Any Body Can Sit and Be Fit was commissioned by the Illinois State Medical Auxiliary for use in nursing homes by the wheelchair-bound or other individuals who find it difficult to stand and do exercise. Flexibility is improved by following the exercises in this 20-minute video.

Forever Fit for 55 and Over provides excellent guidance for improving flexibility and works as a warm-up before aerobic exercise.

Warming Up: The Gentle Exercise Videotape for Formerly Inactive People. This program is designed for people who want to start, or get back to, enjoying regular exercise for fun, healing, and health. It is also useful for people who are overweight.

GOVERNMENT, CONSUMER, AND ADVOCACY GROUPS

Aging in America (AIA), 1500 Pelham Parkway, South, Bronx NY 10461, (312) 545-6900
  A $2.5 million budget allows this organization to conduct research and provide services to professionals in gerontology. The main objectives of the AIA are to produce, implement, and share effective and affordable programs and services that improve the quality of life for older Americans. The AIA also provides a telephone information, referral, and advocacy service. The AIA publishes *Aging in America/ Morningside House Newsletter* and publishes a brochure outlining the organization's numerous programs.
American Association of Homes for the Aging

(AAHA), 1129 20th Street, NW, Suite 400, Washington, DC 20036, (202) 296-5960

This association works to identify and solve problems and to protect and advance the interests of the residents served. The AAHA believes that long-term care should be geared toward individual needs in nursing homes, independent living situations, and community-based care programs. The AAHA publishes *American Association of Homes for the Aging Publications Catalog* and other material.

American Association of Retired Persons (AARP), 3200 East Carson Street, Lakewood, CA 90712, (202) 872-4700

The AARP is the nation's largest group for retired citizens. There are 4,000 local chapters totaling more than 30 million members age 50 and over. The organization provides extensive information and support services for its members at substantial discounts. Services include low-rate credit cards, the AARP Motoring Plan, pharmaceuticals, group health insurance, and more. The AARP also provides information on preparing tax returns, estate planning, health issues, retirement homes, and other concerns of seniors. It provides free publications and lists of service groups. The AARP also lobbies Congress to further the rights, services, and protections for older Americans. The AARP's publications include the *AARP Bulletin* and *Modern Maturity*.

American Health Foundation (AHF), 320 East 43rd Street, New York, NY 10017, (212) 953-1900

The AHF is devoted to promoting preventive medicine. The foundation conducts research into environmental carcinogens and nutrition, provides clinical research and service for adults and children, educates laypeople and medical personnel in the principles of preventive medicine, and investigates the costs of disease and compares them with the costs of preventive approaches. The AHF publishes *Health Letter* bimonthly.

American Longevity Association (ALA), 1000 West Carson Street, Torrance, CA 90509, (213) 553-2764

The ALA is comprised of scientists and laypeople interested in the acceleration of research programs that study the mechanisms of aging, arteriosclerosis, heart attack, stroke, use of artificial hearts, cryopreservation of organs, and other areas relevant to longevity. The ALA publishes *Longevity Letter* monthly.

American Senior Citizens Association (ASCA), P.O. Box 41, Fayetteville, NC 28302, (919) 323-3641

The purpose of the ASCA is to promote the physical, mental, emotional, and economic well-being of senior citizens. The association believes that senior citizens have the right to live with competence, security, and dignity. The organization promotes activities that help senior citizens to be active participants in their communities and publishes *Senior Citizens Voice* bimonthly.

American Society on Aging (ASA), 833 Market Street, Suite 512, San Francisco, CA 94103, (415) 543-2617

The ASA works to enhance the well-being of older individuals and to foster unity among those working with and for the elderly. The organization offers continuing education opportunities in aging-related fields for health-care and social service professionals. The ASA produces several publications.

Association of Informed Senior Citizens (AISC), 460 Spring Park Place, Suite 1000, Herndon, VA 22070, (703) 437-7600

The membership of AISC includes individuals who are 55 and older. The association serves as a consumer interest group and disseminates information and published material on services, discounts, and government-funded programs for senior citizens.

Beverly Foundation (BF), 99 South Oakland Avenue, Suite 227, Pasadena, CA 91101, (818) 792-2292

The Beverly Foundation seeks to promote a positive attitude toward and among the elderly. The organization works to create imaginative self-help programs and opportunities for older adults and their communities, as well as programs to improve long-term care systems and methods of care through education, research, and demonstrations. The foundation publishes *Welcome to Our Nursing Home Study Guide*, in addition to books, manuals, guidebooks, and videotapes.

The Center for Social Gerontology (TCSG), 117 N. First Street, Suite 204, Ann Arbor, MI 48104, (313) 665-1126

The purpose of the center is to advance the well-being of older people in the United States through research, education, technical assistance, and training. The TCSG focuses primarily on legal rights and services, guardianship and alternative protective services, and housing for the elderly. The organization maintains a library of volumes, films, and reference material on legal and policy issues. The TCSG publishes numerous reports, audiovisual materials, and manuals, including *A Comprehensive Guide to Legal Assistance for Older Americans.*

Center for the Study of Aging (CSA), 706 Madison Avenue, Albany, NY 12208, (518) 465-6927
The CSA promotes education, research, and training in the field of health fitness for older people. The group includes volunteers and professionals in aging, gerontology, wellness, fitness, and health. The CSA conducts seminars and weekly radio programs and maintains a 5,000-volume library on aging, medicine, physical activity, and sports.

Children of Aging Parents (CAP), 2761 Trenton Road, Levittown, PA 19056, (215) 945-6900
This self-help group is devoted to the education, support, guidance, and development of coping skills of those who care for the elderly. The group provides workshops for community groups and in-house training for social workers and for nurses in hospitals, nursing homes, and rehabilitation centers. The group also provides referrals to appropriate professionals. CAP publishes the bimonthly *CAPSULE,* which reports on CAP programs and concerns of elderly persons and their families. CAP also publishes *How to Start a Self-Help Group for Caregivers, Instant Aging-Sensory Deprivation Manual,* and *Guide to Selecting a Nursing Home.*

Concerned Relatives of Nursing Home Patients (CRNHP), P.O. Box 18820, Cleveland, OH 44118, (216) 321-0403
Membership consists of volunteers, family members, friends, or guardians of nursing home patients. The organization seeks to achieve dignity and comfort for all nursing home patients and monitors quality of care in nursing homes. The CRNHP disseminates information on nursing homes to consumers, advises families and social service workers on nursing home placement, and maintains a library of statistics for consumer use. The group publishes *Insight* bimonthly and *Selecting a Nursing Home.*

Gray Panthers (GP), 311 South Juniper Street, Suite 601, Philadelphia, PA 19107, (215) 545-6555
This group consists of 100 consciousness-raising local groups composed of older adults and young people who work to combat discrimination against persons on the basis of chronological age. The Gray Panthers believe that both the old and the young have much to contribute to make our society more just and humane. The Gray Panthers maintain research files, offer an information and referral service, and publish newsletters, manuals, and books.

High Blood Pressure Information Center (HBPIC), 120/80 National Institutes of Health, Bethesda, MD 20205, (301) 652-7700
The HBPIC provides information on the detection, diagnosis, and management of high blood pressure to consumers and health professionals. The center identifies, collects, organizes, and disseminates information in many formats. Its sources are monographs, journals, newsletters, newspapers, reports, audiovisual tapes, brochures, posters, and contacts with other health agencies and clearinghouses. The center also provides reference and referral services, consultants, a speakers' register, packets, searches in the Center's data base and resources of other libraries and clearinghouses, and referrals to other sources.

International Senior Citizens Association (ISCA), 1102 South Crenshaw Boulevard, Los Angeles, CA 90019, (213) 857-6434
ISCA's membership includes individuals 50 years of age and older and professional groups. The organization provides coordination on the international level to safeguard the needs and interests of senior citizens worldwide, establishes the means of communication among older citizens for educational and cultural developments, and acts as a forum through which older persons may contribute to world betterment.

National Council of Senior Citizens (NCSC), 925 15th Street, NW, Washington DC 20005, (202) 347-8800
This organization, founded in 1961, has a combined membership of over 4.5 million individuals and encourages legislators and the general population to support Medicare, increase Social Security benefits, improve recreational, educational, and health programs, reduce the costs of pharmaceuticals, and provide for better housing and other programs to aid senior Americans. The NCSC publishes *Senior Citizens News* monthly and distributes news updates, films, reports, and other materials.

National Council on the Aging (NCOA), 600 Maryland Avenue, SW, West Wing, Suite 100, Washington DC 20024, (202) 479-1200

The NCOA was founded in 1950 and cooperates with other organizations to promote concern for older people and develop methods and resources for meeting their medical, social, and housing needs. The NCOA conducts research and demonstration programs on issues of interest to older citizens such as training and job placement, access to health and social services, and services for the frail elderly living at home. The organization maintains a 14,000-volume library on the psychological, economic, and social aspects of aging. The NCOA publishes several books, newsletters, pamphlets, and brochures on all aspects of aging.

National Senior Citizens Law Center (NSCLC), 1052 West Sixth Street, Suite 700, Los Angeles, CA 90017, (213) 482-3550

The NSCLC is a legal services support center specializing in the legal problems of the elderly. It acts as an advocate on behalf of the poor, elderly client in litigation and administrative affairs. The center maintains a library and publishes *Newsletter* weekly, *Nursing Home Law Letter* monthly, and several handbooks, guides, and testimonies.

Older Women's League (OWL), 730 11th Street, NE, Suite 300, Washington, DC 20001, (202) 783-6686

OWL consists of middle-aged and older women and persons of any age who support issues of concern to mid-life and older women. The league addresses access to health-care insurance, support for family caregivers, reform of Social Security, access to jobs and pensions for older women, effects of budget cuts on women, and ways to maintain self-sufficiency throughout life. The league publishes several newsletters and produces videotapes.

Index

Boldface page numbers refer to the pages in which the terms are defined.